Exploring Your Options: Making Informed Decisions About Hormones

EXPLORING YOUR OPTIONS: MAKING INFORMED DECISIONS ABOUT HORMONES

Practical Answers for Women in Pre-, Peri- and Postmenopause

Carol Uebelacker, M.D.

iUniverse, Inc.
New York Lincoln Shanghai

Exploring Your Options: Making Informed Decisions About Hormones

Practical Answers for Women in Pre-, Peri- and Postmenopause

iUniverse, Inc.

For information address:
iUniverse, Inc.
2021 Pine Lake Road, Suite 100
Lincoln, NE 68512
www.iuniverse.com

The suggestions in this book are not meant to be a substitute for a careful medical evaluation by your doctor. This book is intended for educational purposes and the use of the information presented should be used with discretion.

ISBN: 0-595-30878-3

Printed in the United States of America

To My Family

CONTENTS

▼

PART III: STAYING HEALTHY AT THIS STAGE IN YOUR LIFE

PART I

▼

ONE SIZE DOES NOT FIT ALL

The Women's Health Initiative study (WHI) and Britain's Million Women study, both designed to look at health effects from combined estrogen-progestin therapy and estrogen alone, showed a statistically higher risk of breast cancer, heart problems, Alzheimer's disease, and stroke from drugs commonly prescribed for middle-aged women. The interpretation of the studies and statistics is what is really important. Women need to ask, "How do the studies apply to me as an individual?"

Unfortunately, the press (and some doctors) lump all hormones into a single category and rarely think beyond a one-size-fits-all-approach to hormone replacement therapy.

The sloppy media reports leave women feeling panicky about hormone therapy in general. At a time when there are more hormone options than ever (including human identical hormones and others that have not been added to the large studies), the media have routinely put together clumsy stories that generate fear.

The last decade has brought a heightened interest in female reproductive functions and, it is hoped, this trend will continue. What is important to understand is that there have been very few large-scale studies done on human-identical hormones and other hormone preparations. The studies that have attracted media attention are narrow because they focus on Prempro and Premarin alone. This book is aimed at examining several issues surrounding hormone therapy including natural alternatives. Until the large research institutions include a broader range of hormone replacement products in their studies, it will be up to women and their physicians to assemble information that can be used to make informed choices.

CHAPTER 1

▼

THE WHI STUDY
EXPLAINED

On July 9, 2002, when data from the Women's Health Initiative study was released, a storm of news stories broke that spread fear and panic among millions of American women. The media reported that a very large medical study (WHI) had demonstrated that hormone replacement therapy (HRT) not only fails to protect postmenopausal women from heart disease, but also *increases* their risks of heart disease, stroke, breast cancer, and Alzheimer's disease and, furthermore, does nothing for their quality of life.

The news stories about the dangers of hormone therapy continue to hit hard. Doctors were immediately put on the front line and were expected to answer tough questions, since the results from such a high-profile study seemed definitive. The Women's Health Initiative study, started in 1991 by the National Institutes of Health, is designed to study more than 160,000 postmenopausal women ages 50 to 70. The $725 million, 15-year project is actually comprised of several studies at 40 research institutions and more than 150 spin-off studies.

THE STUDY THAT CAUSED PANIC

The results of medical studies rarely make their way to the national media. However, the WHI study was not only large, but it was also organized by a high-profile government organization. When the Prempro arm of the study was halted several years ahead of schedule, the news was startling because Prempro was supposed to prevent life-threatening diseases, not cause them.

Unexpected Increase in Heart Attacks and Cancer

More than 16,000 women who participated in the Prempro arm of the WHI study volunteered for a combination therapy consisting of estrogen and progestin (Premarin and Provera). Some of the women were assigned to randomly receive the hormone combination and some were given a placebo or dummy pill, making the study a double-blind randomly controlled trial. The women would be followed for eight years and monitored for heart attacks, strokes, blood clots, hip fractures, and colon cancer along with other health parameters. A safety board was given the task of analyzing data to ensure that the study would be stopped before its scheduled ending in 2005

- if there was such a clear benefit to the hormone group that it would be unethical to withhold the drug from the control group, and/or

- if the risks of hormone therapy outweighed the benefits so much that women who received the hormones should stop taking theirs.

Another group of women who had had hysterectomies were given Premarin alone. This part of the study, which looks at the long-term use of estrogen alone, is not yet complete. So far, the women who are part of the Premarin-alone study have not shown the same supposedly adverse effects as Prempro.

In late 1999, the monitoring board saw an unexpected statistical increase in blood clots and heart attacks among women on Premarin and Provera, and by the spring of 2002, they saw an increased risk of developing breast cancer. As a result, the monitoring board brought the study to a halt. Although the women on hormone therapy showed fewer hip fractures, the benefit did not outweigh the risk. The question women now need to ask is, "How do these statistical risks apply to me?"

ERRONEOUS INTERPRETATION BY THE MEDIA

At first glance the WHI study seemed to dominate all other studies because of its size. Not only would researchers track 160,000 ethnically diverse women but they would also draw blood samples from the participants at the beginning of the study and one year later. The physical storage requirements for the blood samples challenge the imagination but provide clues about the magnitude of the study. The samples have been stored in 25-cubic-foot freezers and all 114 of the freezers are in Rockville, Maryland. In contrast, an average household refrigerator is 8 to 10 cubic feet. Because the samples have been subdivided into smaller samples, the freezers contain 4 million vials. The samples will be used in spin-off studies for years to come.

Although large in scope, the WHI study has several design flaws. The flaws, combined with the media's misinterpretation of results, may seriously jeopardize future studies of estrogen action. One of the most disturbing outcomes of the study has been the media feeding frenzy that followed the halt in the Prempro arm of the trial. Nearly every report was negative. Sensational headlines included:

WERE WOMEN USED AS GUINEA PIGS IN HORMONE REPLACEMENT THERAPY TREATMENTS?

THE RISE AND FALL OF HORMONE REPLACEMENT THERAPY RANKS AMONG THE BIGGEST MEDICAL MISTAKES IN HISTORY

PILLS DO MORE HARM THAN GOOD

The media companies that delivered these stories were high-profile news organizations such as CNN and ABC News. None of the companies seemed to do extensive research into the issues surrounding hormone replacement therapy. They all seemed to dwell on death and disease. The media coverage was a mile wide and an inch deep. It will now be up to women and their doctors to piece together a more accurate picture of estrogen.

Fortunately, many Americans are aware that the media is self-serving and full of alarmist reports. Many doctors in menopausal care have since published articles and statements to try to reverse the tide of erroneous interpretation caused by the news media.

WHI Backpeddling

Now that the bombshell has been dropped, WHI researchers are backpeddling somewhat. For example, Gloria Bachman, M.D., associate director of women's health for University of Medicine and Dentistry of New Jersey-Robert Wood Johnson Medical School and a coinvestigator on WHI, likens the issue of risks versus benefits to driving a car. "We could be in a fatal accident but if the car is the best way of getting from A to B, then we don't outlaw cars. We try to minimize the risks by wearing seat belts or following speed limits." In an interview with Maryann B. Brinley, a reporter for *Healthstate* magazine, Dr. Bachman described the coronary heart disease numbers in the Prempro study as "lower than what was expected in the general population," adding that "women did very well in terms of cardiovascular disease."

FLAWS IN THE WHI STUDY

The media's overzealous quest for sensational news stories isn't the only reason there have been erroneous interpretations of the Prempro study. For those who do their homework, the subject of hormones is extremely complex. Hormones are part of the body's vast endocrine system, the communication system of glands, hormones, and cellular receptors that control the body's internal functions.

Although it's not necessary to understand everything there is to know about hormones, knowledge is power. The subject of hormones affects 50 million American women, and understanding the flaws in the WHI study will help women evaluate future studies of estrogen action. Important talking points include the following:

Single Estrogen-Progestin Formulation

The combined estrogen-progestin drug used in the trial was Prempro, donated by Wyeth Pharmaceuticals. The WHI results apply only to one formulation. Unfavorable findings were only discovered in the Prempro, or combined estrogen-progestin arm of the study. The estrogen-only arm is being allowed to continue, so it is likely that benefits are being seen. News stories have conveniently overlooked this point.

Women who have followed this story in the press will note that no reporter has asked if the synthetic progestin is offsetting the benefits of the Premarin. If the only difference between the two studies is the presence or absence of Provera (medroxy-progesterone acetate, or MPA), it may be that the problem lies with the MPA.

Critics who see flaws in the WHI study also point out that human-identical hormones are entirely missing from the study. Human-identical, or bio-identical, hormones and other products are used by a growing number of women and will be presented later in this book. Many people have pointed out that a trial that includes human-identical hormones should have an additional arm:

- Placebo control

- Estrogen only (various brands and formulations)

- Combined estrogen-progestin (various brands and formulations)

- Alternative human-identical hormones

In an essay on his Web site, Alan M. Altman, M.D., assistant clinical professor of obstetrics, gynecology and reproductive biology at Harvard Medical School, wrote:

*The WHI study was **not** a study of HRT. It was a study of a specific product called Prempro, a product that combines horse-derived estrogen and an extremely potent progestin called MPA in a single pill. A product that is totally different from the 40-plus other presently available HRT products in the US.*

*Those of us who specialize in peri and postmenopausal care have been well aware over the past 10 to 15 years that MPA, the synthetic progestin used in Prempro, is too strong and can act to reduce many of the benefits estrogens may provide. This is the principle reason so many other natural and synthetic progestins have been developed to allow avoidance of MPA use in HRT. These newer and safer progestins have been widely used in Europe, where they use little, if any, MPA, and have been used here in the US by practitioners who understand the differences and how to make most optimum use of these options. **It is thoroughly inappropriate to extend the WHI study results to any other kind of HRT.***

Many of the Women Studied Were Not Healthy

The authors of the WHI study have made the claim that the women studied were healthy and that the goal of the study was to monitor the effects of hormones on diseases of the aging such as cardiovascular disease and cancer. In spite of the authors' claim, a large number of the women were not healthy:

- 35% were treated for hypertension
- 35% were overweight
- 34% were obese
- 4% were diabetic
- 12.5% had elevated cholesterol levels requiring medication
- 6.9% used statins (anticholesterol drugs)

Thirty Percent of the Women Studied Were Over 70

The goal of the WHI study was to assess the effect of hormone therapy on the diseases of aging, not on short-term relief of hot flashes and other menopausal symptoms, for which hormone therapy is often used. The average age of the women studied was 63, and thirty percent of the women were over 70. Most critics feel the study's 16,000 participants were too old to provide relevant information about menopause. The average age at menopause in the United States is 51. Dr. Frederick Naftolin, head of the Yale Center for Reproductive Biology in New Haven, Connecticut has said, "It's probably too late for estrogen to protect against heart disease by the seventh decade of life. The WHI results aren't applicable to patients complaining of menopause symptoms."

The women recruited were 50 to 79 years of age, and screening for the existence of cardiovascular disease was accomplished with a questionnaire. Because of their age, the pool of participants carried a very high probability of preexisting cardiovascular disease.

RELATIVE VS. ABSOLUTE RISK

It is important for women to understand that the news stories containing details about the Women's Health Initiative study focused on the more dramatic *relative risk* findings rather than the absolute risks. The increases in the relative risks of coronary heart disease, breast cancer, stroke, and pulmonary blood clots were widely quoted in the media. The relative figures show alarmingly high numbers. In *absolute* terms, these numbers are very small and are much less alarming:

Absolute Risk of Estrogen Plus Progestin Therapy

Disease	Cases per 10,000 Women on HRT For 1 Year	Cases per 10,000 Women *on No HRT For 1 Year*
Coronary Heart Disease	37	30
Breast Cancer	38	30
Stroke	29	21
Blood clots	34	16

Where do the numbers come from?

Relative and absolute risk are labels used by research scientists who compare data. These terms have been explained on the National Heart, Lung and Blood Institute's Web site (www.nhlbi.nih.gov) using breast cancer rates as an example.

After five years, the estrogen-plus-progestin arm of the WHI study had 166 cases of breast cancer among the estrogen plus progestin users compared with 124 in the placebo group. Because there were more women in the hormone group (8,506) compared with the placebo group (8,102), these figures were converted to rates per 10,000 per year in order to compare the data. The rate of breast cancer was 38 per 10,000 women in the hormone group compared to 30 per 10,000 in the placebo group. These numbers can also be expressed as 38/30, which equals 1.26. In other words, in relative terms, 38 is 26 percent larger than 30.

However, in any single year, in a group of 10,000 women, 8 additional women will develop breast cancer if they are estrogen-plus-progestin users (Figure 1). This smaller, much less alarming, number is calculated by dividing 8/10,000, which equals .08.

At a scientific workshop on menopausal hormone therapy sponsored by the National Institutes of Health, Dr. Otis Brawley of Emory University called relative risk findings "scientific salesmanship." He said, "If you want to emphasize the findings, use relative risk." And that's just what the media did. It should also be noted that the 33 percent reduction in hip fractures and 37 percent reduction in colorectal cancer was de-emphasized and almost ignored.

Figure 1

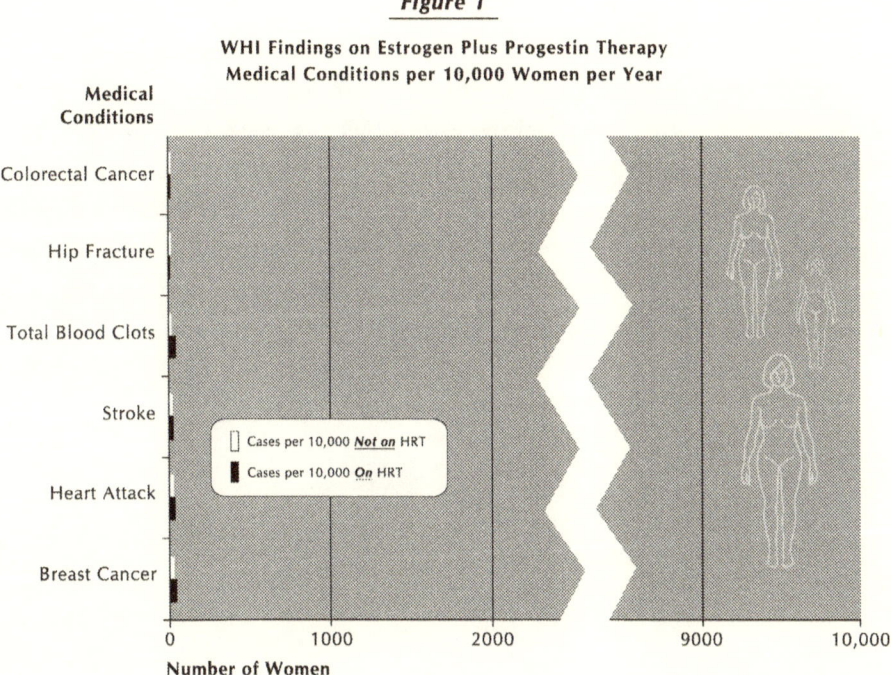

WHI Findings on Estrogen Plus Progestin Therapy
Medical Conditions per 10,000 Women per Year

THE NEED FOR CONTINUED RESEARCH

In the next 20 years, approximately 40 million women will enter menopause. The medical consequences of a one-size-fits-all approach to solving the problems of menopause have been brought to light by the WHI study. It is worth noting, however, that

• Only one brand of hormones was studied

• The actual risk to the individual is naturally low whether a woman is on hormones or not

- The estrogen-alone arm of the WHI study is ongoing, indicating that benefits have already been seen

- The study has numerous selection flaws

As a result, women often need to research the subject of hormones on their own.

My purpose in writing this book is to help women find the information they need to make informed decisions. Although science knows more about hormones than ever before, the subject is large and complex and there is still more to learn. In addition, sex hormones are surprisingly interconnected to a multitude of other functions. The road to health requires good health practices, and there are no magic pills. Nature likes balance and when the hormones in a woman's body are out of balance, it is usually a signal that raw materials are needed for fine-tuning.

CHAPTER 2

▼

BALANCED HORMONE HEALTH

The study of women's hormones includes several cutting-edge physiologic issues, including cardiology, sugar and bone metabolism, cognition, mood disorders, and memory. Because sex hormones control more than the reproductive cycle, this chapter includes details about sex hormones as well as other hormones that play an important role in female hormone health.

A book about hormones would not be complete if it did not have a review of what takes place during menstruation. Although every woman is aware of what takes place in her body each month, a review is helpful because menopause represents the end of a woman's hormone cycles. Learning these details is particularly important at a time when the media over-generalizes about hormones and presents insufficient information in their news reports. Women who possess more than a surface understanding of health issues will be able to identify poorly written reports that do nothing more than spread fear.

HORMONES IN A WOMAN'S BODY

If you open a biology book or encyclopedia and look up *Endocrine System*, you'll see that the ovaries are part of a vast network that controls functions in a woman's body. Books that provide details about ovarian function usually contain a compartmentalized list of female hormones and the glands where they are usually made.

To say hormones are usually made in the glands is a little misleading because they are also made in cells where they can be synthesized from other hormones. The liver plays an important role in this process because hormones are made from cholesterol and cholesterol is produced in the liver (see: "Cholesterol is a Hormone Precursor")

Female Hormones

Sex hormones are considered steroid hormones, a category that also includes many metabolic hormones. The three main categories of hormones include the following:

Steroid hormones
This class includes metabolic and sex hormones that are lipid like and are formed from cholesterol (Note: This is a key point that will be discussed later in the book). Hormones from the adrenal cortex and gonads are included in this category.

Peptide hormones
These hormones are formed from short amino acid chains. Hormones formed in the hypothalamus and pituitary fit into this category.

Amine hormones
These hormones are derived from the amino acid tyrosine. Adrenal medulla and thyroid hormones are included in this category.

Although this section may seem a lot like biology class and somewhat boring, women who read articles about hormone replacement therapy should know the names and functions of the different estrogens. All too often, a reporter will refer to *estrogen* and not specify the particular estrogen. As you will see in this chart, the various estrogens have different functions.

Hormone	Principal Gland	Description
Estrogens:	Ovaries	A class of hormones that includes many different subcategories. The major estrogens include estrone, estradiol and estriol. Estrogens promote breast development and cause cyclic changes in a woman's body. **Note: Each of the three types of estrogens have a different function in a woman's body. Articles in the press can be misleading without the specific reference to the type of estrogen.**
• **Estrone (E1)**		An inactive form of estrogen that is produced in body fat and is considered to be the dominant form of estrogen after menopause.
• **Estradiol (E2)**		An active form of estrogen produced in the ovaries as well as several other sites in the body such as the bones, the blood vessels, and the brain.
• **Estriol (E3)**		A benign form of estrogen that is predominant in the womb. According to Dr. Jonathan Wright, who created a hormone supplement called Tri-Est, the body's pattern of circulating estrogen is 10–20% estrone, 10–20% estradiol and 60–80% estriol.
Follicle-stimulating Hormone (FSH)	Pituitary	Hormone produced in the brain that initiates the ovulation cycle and stimulates the production of estrogen in follicles. Follicles are tiny sacs within each ovary. Each follicle contains an egg, and it is thought that women have as many as 500,000 follicles when menstruation begins.

Luteinizing Hormone (LH)	Pituitary	Hormone that stimulates a follicle to release an egg during ovulation. This hormone also stimulates estrogen and progesterone production in the corpus luteum (egg sac).
Progesterone	Ovaries	The dominant hormone in the second half of a menstrual cycle that is produced by the corpus luteum or empty sac that produced the ovum or egg in a given month.
Testosterone	Ovaries	A hormone produced in both men and women. This hormone maintains a woman's libido and contributes to bone strength.

HORMONE CYCLES DURING MENSTRUATION

The hormones that govern the menstrual cycle are produced by the pituitary gland and ovaries. The cycle is divided into four phases and occurs approximately every 28 days. However, it can span anywhere from 20 to 40 days in some women.

Day 1–5, Menstrual Bleeding

Bleeding marks the first day of the menstrual cycle. Approximately 5 days later, the bleeding subsides. Menstruation occurs in response to a drop in the level of progesterone from the previous cycle (Figure 2).

Day 6–13, Follicular or Proliferative Phase

The second phase of the menstrual cycle, which lasts until day 13, is called the follicular or proliferative phase. The ovary begins the egg maturation process in response to the follicle-stimulating hormone and the luteinizing hormone from the pituitary gland (Figure 2). Ten to twenty eggs begin to develop within follicles inside the ovaries, but only one egg will reach maturity. Follicles are clusters of cells surrounding a developing egg. The developing follicles release estrogen that stimulates the lining of the uterus or endometrium. Growth occurs or proliferation occurs in the lining in preparation for a fertilized embryo.

Day 14, Ovulation Phase

Ovulation occurs in the third phase in response to high levels of estrogen that trigger a surge in the luteinizing hormone that will cause a dominant follicle to release an egg. Ovulation usually occurs on day 14 (Figure 2).

Day 14, Luteal, Secretory, or Postovulatory Phase

The fourth phase usually lasts from days 15–28 (Figure 2). An empty follicle, now called the corpus luteum, releases the hormone progesterone, which prepares the uterus for an embryo. Acting as an antagonist to the hormone estrogen that stimulates cell growth, progesterone halts further ovulation during the second half of the menstrual cycle. If pregnancy does not occur, a fall in progesterone initiates the beginning of a new cycle. If pregnancy does occur, progesterone levels remain high and the endometrium is not shed.

CHOLESTEROL IS A HORMONE PRECURSOR

Sex hormones are produced in the body in more than one metabolic pathway. Through an impressive system of checks and balances, hormones can be used to suppress the production of other hormones if, for example, a particular hormone is out of balance. Hormones can also be converted to other hormones if there is a shortage.

Estrogens and progesterone are made in a woman's ovaries between puberty and menopause. After menopause, the ovaries may still produce low levels of hormones supplemented by hormones produced in the adrenal glands. As a result, it is important for a woman to maintain healthy adrenal glands after menopause.

Figure 2

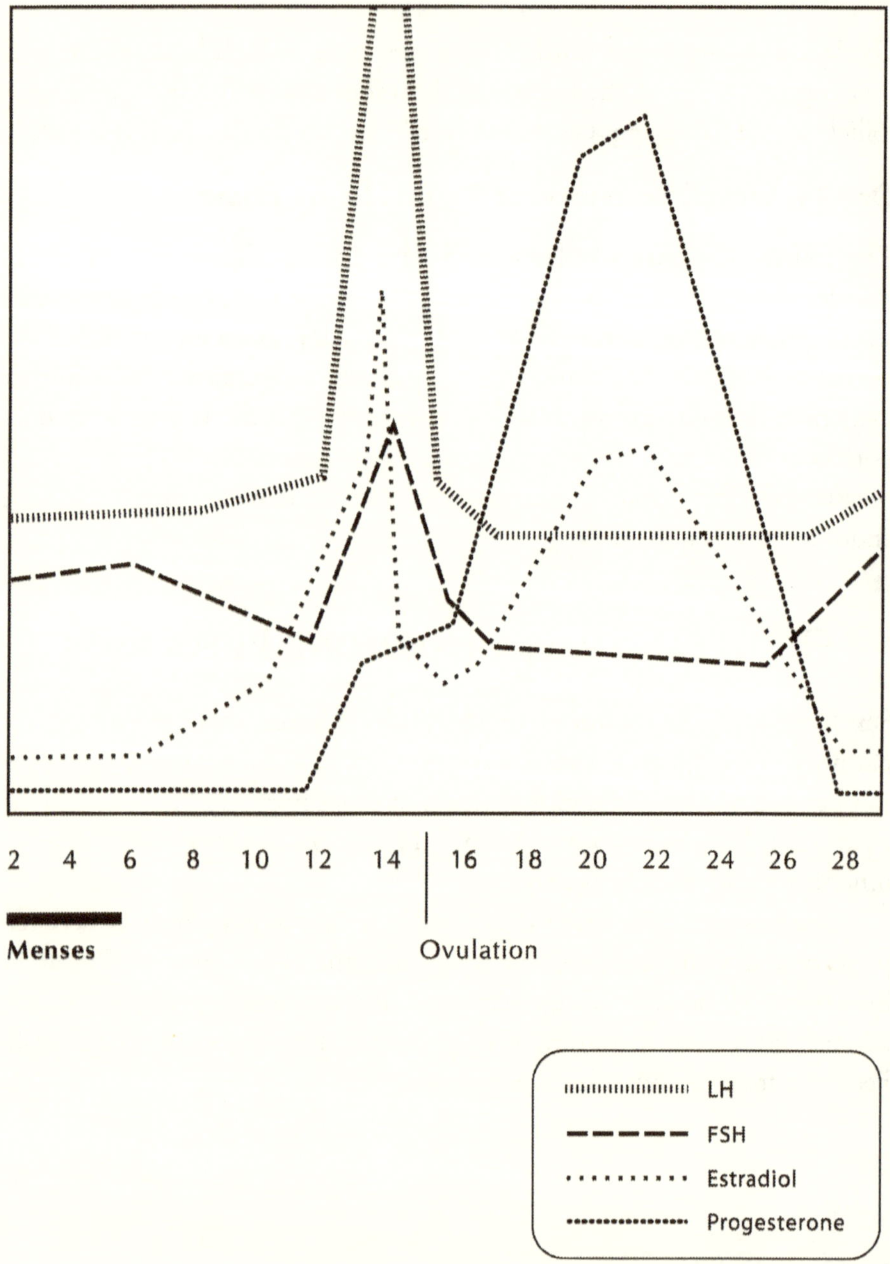

2   4   6   8   10   12   14   16   18   20   22   24   26   28

Menses   Ovulation

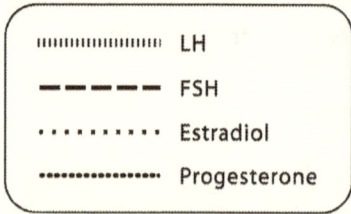

ⅰⅰⅰⅰⅰⅰⅰⅰⅰ	LH
– – – – –	FSH
·········	Estradiol
···········	Progesterone

The diagram that follows is a simplified illustration of hormone production in the adrenal cortex (Figure 3). From this diagram, known as the steroid hormone cascade, readers will be able to see that

- Cholesterol is an important precursor or ancestor molecule that is used to produce a range of steroid or sex hormones.

- Pregnenolone is the first molecule to be produced from cholesterol. The rate at which the adrenal cortex makes pregnenolone will determine the rate at which other steroid hormones will be created.

- From pregnenolone, the next step creates either progesterone or dehydroepiandrosterone (DHEA). DHEA is used to make estrogen or androgens (male hormones that are also present in a woman's body).

- Progesterone can be used as a building block for estrogen. As a result, some doctors like to recommend progesterone as a supplement when there is a hormone problem because it gives the body many options about what to do next.

- Estradiol has more than one metabolic pathway. Notice that the male hormone testosterone can be converted into estradiol, which is a female hormone.

- When the body is under high stress, the body will produce cortisol at the expense of the other hormones. High stress means greatly reduced reproductive/sex hormones. Dr. Nicholas Perricone, author of *The Wrinkle Cure* calls cortisol the "death hormone." Even though it is an essential hormone used to combat stress, it has a lot of negative side effects. High levels of cortisol can break down muscle tissue, thin our skin, decalcify our bones, and elevate our blood sugar.

Steroid Hormone Cascade in the Adrenal Cortex

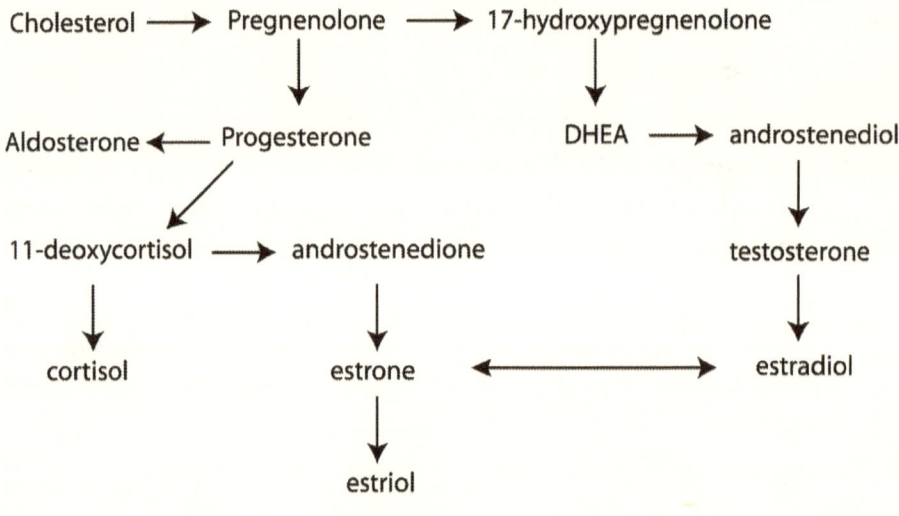

Figure 3.

CONNECTIONS BETWEEN HORMONE SYSTEMS

Few books provide an accurate view of how the ovaries and sex hormones are part of an interrelated whole or the balanced "system" that controls every function in the body. To illustrate the connections between different hormone systems, consider the following:

Gland	Related Functions
Pancreas	Insulin released from the pancreas serves to lower glucose levels in the blood by moving it into muscle cells where it is burned to provide energy or by moving it into fat cells where it is stored for future energy needs. A condition known as insulin resistance occurs when insulin is no longer able to move glucose into cells. Most often caused by genetics or eating excessive amounts of sugar, insulin resistance often leads to diabetes and heart disease. Chronically high insulin is associated with polycystic ovary syndrome (PCOS) or an abnormality in the production of estrogen and progesterone causing ovulation to stop (anovulatory cycle). Insulin also causes the ovaries to produce male hormones called androgens, causing weight gain around the waist.
Adrenal	In premenopause, periods do not occur when there's not enough progesterone (because of a reduced number of follicles and associated progesterone production in the corpus luteum or egg sac). In older women, progesterone is produced in the adrenal glands, which are a backup system for progesterone production. At menopause, if a woman's adrenal glands are healthy, they can produce a follicular level of progesterone.
Thyroid	Estrone, the estrogen usually found in heavy women, can inhibit the thyroid gland. At menopause, the ovaries stop producing estrogen and progesterone, but continue to produce androstenedione, a male hormone that is converted to estrogen in fat cells. In younger women, hypothyroidism or low thyroid can cause menstrual problems such as PMS and heavy periods, fertility problems, stiffness of joints, and muscular cramps. An underactive thyroid decreases the metabolism, which secondarily decreases the likelihood of ovulation.

Given these interrelated connections to other glands in the endocrine system, it's difficult to understand why it has taken researchers over 50 years to realize that

- There's a delicate balance required in the body's hormone system.

- A one-size-fits-all approach to hormone replacement therapy does not work.

- Sex hormones need to be considered in relationship to each other and in relationship to other hormones produced in the body.

PART II

▼

THE STAGES OF MENOPAUSE AND WHAT WE KNOW ABOUT THEM

Premenopause

Women in this stage are still ovulating but show signs of a decline in ovarian hormones as early as their mid-thirties.

Perimenopause

Women in this stage may still be menstruating and have menopausal symptoms, but they're no longer ovulating regularly.

Menopause

Menopause is official when you have had no periods for twelve months.

Postmenopause

Postmenopause can be used to describe the stage in a woman's life after menopause is official.

CHAPTER 3

▼

HORMONE IMBALANCE BEFORE MENOPAUSE

There is a quiet revolution taking place in women's health care that involves a holistic approach to solving hormone imbalances *before* menopause even begins. If hormone balancing in younger women were part of a medical breakthrough in tweaking the body's endocrine system, it might be good news. However, the truth is that the imbalances that exist may be caused by 70 years of industrialization—and the implications are hair raising.

Only a small percentage of physicians seem to be noticing what is taking place. The doctor witnesses who are taking note live in highly industrialized countries where increasing numbers of women in *all age groups* are experiencing hormone disruptions. The evidence in our midst includes the following:

Early Onset of Puberty

The age at which young girls reach puberty continues to drop. A recent study published in the *Journal of Pediatrics* reveals that one in every seven

Caucasian girls and one in every two African American girls develop breasts or pubic hair before the age of eight.

Endometriosis

Endometriosis, an extremely painful disease that afflicts women from age 20 to 70, is on the rise. The pain is caused by uterine or endometrial tissue that grows in other areas of the body. During a woman's menstrual cycle the tissue bleeds with hormonal changes in the cycle as if it were inside the uterus. Endometriosis has been linked to dioxin, a chemical found increasingly in underwater sediment and in fish. In studies done on rhesus monkeys at the University of South Florida, 79 percent of the females in the colony that were exposed to dioxin developed endometriosis.

Uterine Fibroids

Researchers now estimate that 70 percent of women have fibroids. However, symptoms occur in only 25 percent of women. Uterine fibroids consisting of muscle and connective tissue, are solid benign tumors that are found within the uterus or attached to the uterine wall. Fibroids occur as long as a woman is menstruating and shrink after menopause.

Polycystic Ovarian Syndrome (PCOS)

PCOS was first described as an infertility problem in 1935, but it is now recognized as a complex endocrine disorder affecting 6 to 10 percent of women. Critical complications include insulin resistance as well as an increased risk of cardiovascular disease and breast cancer. Symptoms include irregular or absent menstrual cycles, high blood pressure, acne, elevated insulin levels, insulin resistance or diabetes, infertility, excess hair on the face and body, thinning of the scalp hair (alopecia), and weight problems or obesity that is centered around a woman's midsection.

Breast Cancer

In 1960, the chances of a woman developing breast cancer during her lifetime was one in twenty. Today the chances are an alarming one in eight.

MAJOR FEMALE HORMONES

Although it sounds like school, let's revisit what we know about women's major hormones:

Estrogen

Given that estrogen is a class of hormones and not an individual hormone, it is helpful to review the characteristics of the three major estrogens, starting with the most potent:

Estradiol (E2)

Estradiol is the predominant estrogen prior to menopause. It is mostly produced in the ovaries and is known for its ability to stimulate the growth and multiplication of cells. One of its primary functions is to stimulate the regrowth of the uterine lining in the first half of the menstrual cycle. Prior to ovulation, a surge of estradiol will be needed for ovulation to occur. In fact, ovulation will be dependent on an estrogen threshold that will trigger a surge of luteinizing hormone. When this surge occurs, an egg will burst through the ovarian wall. After this takes place, the egg moves into the pelvic cavity and then moves into the fallopian tubes. At this point, the remains of the ruptured follicle will begin secreting progesterone. Key points to know about estradiol include:

- Estradiol is three times more potent than estrone and ten times more potent than estriol.

- Estradiol is responsible for a regrowth of the uterine lining because of its proliferative effect on cell growth.

- High levels of estradiol are associated with a risk of breast cancer and endometrial cancer.

- Estradiol's growth effect is offset by progesterone.

- The ratio of estradiol to estrone in premenopause is approximately greater than one, which means there is more estradiol than estrone in premenopause.

Estrone (E1)

Estrone is the predominant estrogen after menopause. Although some estrone is produced in the ovaries, it is primarily assembled in fat tissue with the help of an enzyme called aromatase. The building blocks used to form estrone are androgens, the male hormones made in the adrenal glands (androstenedione and testosterone). This process is known as the aromatase pathway, and it also assembles estradiol molecules from estrone (see Figure 3 in Chapter 2). Because estrone is primarily assembled in fat tissue, estrone levels are high in women who are heavy. Key points to know about estrone include the following:

- Estrone is associated with menopause because it is principally manufactured after ovarian decline. When the ovaries slow down, estrone is made via the aromatase pathway.

- High levels of estrone are associated with fat that accumulates around a woman's waist. This distribution of fat can be described in terms of a waist-to-hip ratio found by dividing a woman's waist measurement by her hip measurement. Prior to menopause, a woman's waist-to-hip ratio is supposed to be less than .8. As fat gets distributed at the waist, this ratio is larger than .8. For example:

Waist	Hip	Waist-to-Hip Ratio
26 inches	36 inches.	26/36 = .72
28 inches	36 inches	28/36 = .77
30 inches	36 inches	30/36 = .83
32 inches	36 inches	32/36 = .88

- In heavy women, the ratio of estradiol to estrone is less than one, which means there is less estradiol than estrone. High levels of estrone are associated with diabetes, heart attacks, and breast and uterine cancer.

Estriol (E3)

Estriol is the weakest of the principal estrogens. Scientists are not sure how estriol is made in the body. Some feel it is a metabolite formed when estrone and estadiol are broken down. Others feel it is converted from androstenedione and estrone in the ovaries and adrenals. During pregnancy, the levels of estriol are very high in the womb. As a result, it is an estrogen that has been associated with pregnancy. Key points to know about estriol include these two:

- Estriol has both agonist and antagonist properties. This means it can block activity at an estrogen receptor (antagonist) or promote activity at the receptor (agonist).

- Estriol's benefits have been discovered fairly recently. In a study published in a 1996 issue of the *Journal of the American Medical Association,* estriol was found to be protective against breast and endometrial cancer.

Progesterone

Progesterone plays a vital role in the menstrual cycle because it allows pregnancy to occur. When a ruptured follicle begins secreting progesterone, it will inhibit other eggs from developing and causes the body temperature to rise. It is produced following ovulation by the corpus luteum of a mature ovarian follicle. Smaller amounts are made in the adrenal cortex in both sexes and in the male testes. When progesterone is secreted after ovulation, it causes an increase in blood vessels in the uterine lining in case nutrients are needed to feed a growing fetus. Without fertilization, the progesterone secretion slows down and menstruation begins.

Progesterone also has an important role as a steroid precursor in the synthesis of the adrenal corticosteroid hormones estrogen and testosterone (see Figure 3, Chapter 2). Key points to know about progesterone include:

- Progesterone acts as an antagonist to estrogen. For example, estrogen stimulates cells to grow, and progesterone functions to protect tissues of the body such as the endometrium. It is for this reason that estrogen has been associated with breast and endometrial cancers but progesterone has been known to prevent cancer.

- When women do not ovulate, there is no surge of progesterone because there is no mature egg and no secretion of progesterone from the corpus luteum. However, there is an important balancing act between estrogen and progesterone. It is important to note that ovulation is dependent on an estrogen threshold that will trigger a surge of luteinizing hormone to enable ovulation to occur (see Estrogen, Estradiol in this section).

- Dr. John Lee, author of *What Your Doctor Has Not Told You About Premenopause,* has popularized progesterone as a hormone that may be successful for treating hormone imbalances on its own. In his book *What's Your Menopause Type,* Dr. Joseph Collins describes various "camps" in women's health care that promote "estrogen for all women," "progesterone for all women," and "testosterone for all women." He writes

  Currently, there is tremendous zeal over the use of progesterone. The similarity between the current progesterone craze and the estrogen craze of years gone by is frightening. Success stories are embellished and widely circulated, while side effects and documented problems are ignored. And the next craze looks set to be testosterone which may, in its turn, be hyped as a hormone every woman needs.

  In Collins' view, all three major hormones—estrogen, progesterone, and testosterone—need to be in balance.

- In Dr. Lee's view, women have excess estrogen in their bodies relative to the amount of progesterone, and he calls this a state of "estrogen dominance." This sounds like he's saying all women have excess estrogen, but that is not the case. Although unopposed estrogen and the pervasive amount of environmental estrogen-like substances or xenoestrogens are two prominent themes in all of Lee's books, he acknowledges that women may have an estrogen deficiency. In *What's Your Menopause Type,* Dr. Joseph Collins explains that the condition known as "estrogen dominance" is more accurately described as a "progesterone deficiency."

If you read Dr. Lee's book carefully, you'll see that he says, "A vast majority of women between the ages of forty and seventy are a little bit plump." He calls plumpness nature's mechanism to promote the production of estrogen in fat cells and explains that an estrogen deficiency is found in thin women and not heavy women. It could be that the excess estrogen Lee is referring to is actually estrone (see: Estrogen, Estrone in this chapter). Other authors such as Dr. Elizabeth Vliet and Dr. Edward Klaiber say they often see low estradiol in clinical practice. Could it be that these doctors are all saying the same thing?

Testosterone

Although testosterone is widely considered to be a male hormone, it is also a primary female hormone manufactured in the ovaries. A limited amount of testosterone is also assembled through the aromatase pathway in the fat tissue, liver, skin, and brain (see Figure 3 in Chapter 2). Women's bodies have approximately one tenth the amount of testosterone that is present in a man's body, and the functions are similar. Testosterone increases mental sharpness and energy; relaxes the coronary arteries, thereby allowing increased blood flow to the heart; decreases fat; increases muscle; improves the libido; and increases bone density.

More and more often, doctors are seeing elevated testosterone as one of the symptoms in young women with polycystic ovary syndrome, or PCOS. PCOS is a very serious and complex endocrine disorder that presents itself in childbearing years and earlier. Females with PCOS are heavy, with fat distributed around the waist and upper body. Hormonally, there is usually high testosterone and low estradiol. Besides an excess of testosterone, there can be high levels of other male hormones, namely androstenedione and DHEA. Women with high androgen levels have excess facial and body hair (hirsutism) as well as thinning scalp hair (alopecia). This is sometimes seen in menopausal women with a similar hormone profile. A testosterone hormone imbalance can also cause severe acne, ovarian cysts, insulin resistance combined with glucose intolerance, and irregular menstrual cycles.

In *It's My Ovaries, Stupid!*, Elizabeth Vliet explains that PCOS is often described as an elevated estrogen and elevated androgen syndrome and that this is misleading. She says that the elevated estrogen is actually estrone produced by excess body fat and that estradiol, the most active form of estrogen, is actually lower than expected in women with PCOS.

Dr. Samuel Thatcher, author of *PCOS, The Hidden Epidemic*, says the most common signs of PCOS are obesity, excessive facial and body hair (hirsutism), and lack of timely ovulation. He explains that 95 percent of women who have all three of these symptoms have PCOS. Thatcher also explains that not all PCOS patients are obese, not all are excessively hairy and not all are infertile. He explains that at least 5 percent of all women of reproductive age have some characteristic of PCOS and that some researchers have made a distinction between "PCOS-appearing" ovaries on ultrasound and "true" PCOS. Through pelvic ultrasound, it has been found that 20 to 30% of women of reproductive age have polycystic-appearing ovaries. Thatcher's statistical compilation of a PCOS profile includes the following:

- 20–30% of all women have PCOS changes evident on ultrasound
- 5–10% of all women have elevated androgens and chronic anovulation
- 90% plus of PCOS patients show PCOS on ultrasound
- 40–60% of PCOS patients have weight or obesity problems
- 60–90% of PCOS patients have skin and/or hair problems
- 50–90% of PCOS patients have abnormal ovulation
- 40–80% of PCOS patients have fertility impairment
- 40–80% of PCOS patients demonstrate insulin resistance
- 40% of PCOS patients develop Type 2 diabetes by age 40

In the years leading up to menopause, women can exhibit symptoms that are characteristic of high testosterone as well as low testosterone proving the need for individualized care. According to Dr. Susan Rako, author of *The Hormone of Desire: The Truth About Testosterone, Sexuality and Menopause*, about 50 percent of menopausal women (and some percentage of women in the years leading up to menopause) experience a significant loss of available testosterone with detrimental effects to sexual libido, sensitivity, and response. She explains that not all women are troubled by this. Key points to know about testosterone are as follows:

- Too much testosterone causes acne and increased facial or body hair as well as insulin resistance and an increase in heart disease.

- Because testosterone is a precursor for estrogen, there is a concern that high levels can also contribute to breast cancer.

- A proper amount of testosterone is helpful in maintaining a woman's sex drive, healthy tissues in the vagina, muscle tone and skin collagen.

- Testosterone also has a role in building bone tissue.

HORMONE IMBALANCE AND THE BRAIN

Dr. Edward Klaiber, author of *Hormones and the Mind,* promotes an individualized approach to hormone therapy to treat or prevent depression, mood disorders, cognitive impairment, short-or long-term memory problems, Alzheimer's disease, and dementia as well as sexual disinterest and dysfunction.

In his book, *Hormones and the Mind,* Klaiber also explains that estrogen also increases the density of neurotransmitter receptors on the surface of nerve cells ensuring a "lock and key" fit that is needed for proper neurotransmission and mental well-being. He uses the expression "down rushing elevator" to describe the drop in estrogen levels in a woman's body prior to the onset of menopause that *can cause* psychological and physical havoc.

ARE YOU IN PRE- OR PERIMENOPAUSE?

The decade prior to menopause offers women an opportunity to avert the health problems that are showing up in more and more women. Hormone balancing is the key to endocrine health and practical steps include the following.

Find a Doctor Who Is Up to Date

Hormone balancing is an art that requires well-informed professional supervision. Finding the right doctor may be challenging because most physicians are only aware of what they were taught in medical school. You'll want to find a doctor who is familiar with newer natural hormones available by prescription from compounding pharmacies, along with other prescription formulations. (Note: Compounding pharmacies, listed later in the book, can provide a list of doctors who are familiar with natural hormones.)

Determine if You're Still Ovulating

Women in premenopause are *still* ovulating regularly and women in perimenopause are *no longer* ovulating regularly. By charting your morning basal temperature, you can determine whether you are ovulating. (Note: Menopause, which will be covered later, is official when you have not had your period for a year.)

As described in Chapter 2, the body's progesterone level rises immediately after ovulation and falls just before menstruation begins. Because this change in your progesterone level causes a slight change in body temperature, you can monitor your temperature to determine when progesterone rises and falls. The temperature variation is in tenths of a degree so a digital thermometer is recommended (to see a .4 degree Fahrenheit increase). Expect to pay from five to ten dollars for a digital model in any drugstore. Products labeled "Digital Basal Thermometers" are similar and fall in the same price range.

Fertile women use this technique to determine when they are most likely to get pregnant during their cycle, either to conceive or prevent conception. Your daily temperature recordings can help you determine if you've had an anovulatory cycle (a cycle without ovulation).

When you plot your temperature each morning, you will see your temperature rise at ovulation and remain high until a day or two before the end of the cycle, marking the start of menstruation. If your temperature never rises (indicating no ovulation) or drops several days after ovulation and stays low for days, there is a very good chance that your progesterone levels are low.

When you plot your daily temperature, you'll want to record readings for the entire month. A chart is helpful to record your temperature readings.

For a larger chart with more columns, The Couple to Couple League International provides a free chart download from their Web site at http://www.ccli.org/free/index.shtml. A two-booklet package of fourteen charts is $2.50.

The Couple to Couple League International
P.O. Box 111184
Cincinnati, Ohio 45211-1184
Telephone: (513) 471-2000
www.ccli.org

Steps for Determining Ovulation:

1. Either enlarge the following chart with a photocopier or use the chart as a guide to create your own. Review "Hormone Cycles During Menstruation" in Chapter 2, and recall that Day 1 is considered the day you begin bleeding. Use a pencil to write the date at the top of each column and plot a point near the temperature reading that you need to record.

2. When you awaken, take your temperature immediately. Do not get up out of bed first, even to go to the bathroom, because movement will artificially raise the body temperature. A digital thermometer will beep to alert you when enough time has passed for an accurate reading. It will also display your temperature in tenths of a degree.

3. Try to take your temperature at the same time each morning (or as close as possible).

4. Watch for a rise of .4–1.0 F. (Note: It is normal for body temperature to fluctuate slightly.)

5. For an ovulation-associated increase, you will need to look for an elevated temperature after the lowest temperature point.

6. An elevated temperature should occur on Day 13 or 14. You'll also notice that your temperature remains elevated in the days before your period. If you experience a temperature rise in fewer than ten days, or if you see a drop after a rise, this may be due to anovulation (no ovulation).

Basal Temperature Chart

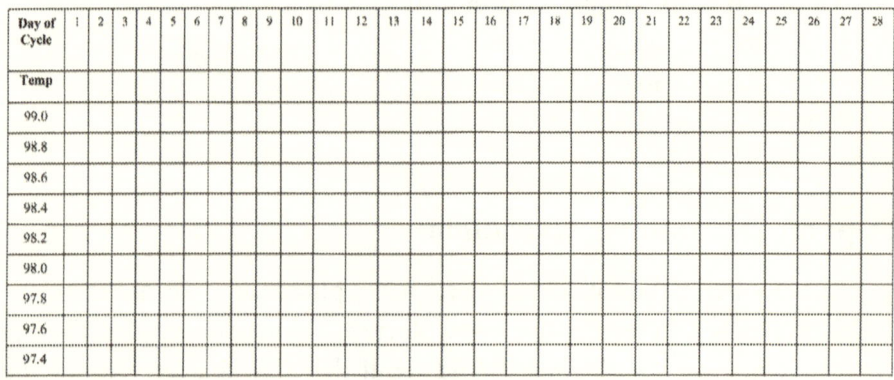

Figure 4.

PLOTTING THE SYMPTOMS OF PREMENOPAUSE

A chart of symptoms will help you understand the patterns of your cycle, and it will help you correlate a possible hormone imbalance. Keeping a record of symptoms will also help you communicate with your doctor. By charting your symptoms, you'll be able to relay exactly what is happening in your body.

Premenopause and Perimenopause Symptom Chart

Month Day				
1				
2				
3				
4				
5				
6				
7				
8				
9				
10				
11				
12				
13				
14				
15				
16				
17				
18				
19				
20				
21				
22				
23				
24				
25				
26				
27				
28				
29				
30				
31				

Figure 5.

Steps for Completing the Chart:

1. Either enlarge the chart above with a photocopier or use it as a guide to create your own.

2. Notice that the numbers in the left column of the chart correspond to the days of the month. Use the space at the top of each column to label the months you are charting. Because you may want to chart your symptoms for several months, you may want to add the year.

3. Use an M to chart the dates you have your menstrual period. For example, if you period starts on the 15th of the month, write an M next to number 15. Fill in more letters depending on the length of your period.

4. Use the following chart as a guide for charting your other symptoms:

Letter	Symptom
M	Menstrual period
B	Breast tenderness
HB	Heavy Bleeding
H	Headaches
C	Cramps
WR	Water Retention
I	Irritability
L	Lethargy

5. (Option) Use the following numbers to chart the severity of your symptoms:

Number	Severity
1	Mild
2	Moderate
3	Severe

CHAPTER 4

▼

BALANCING HORMONES AT PRE-, PERI- AND POSTMENOPAUSE

In the years preceding menopause, you'll most likely experience a decline in one or more of the ovarian hormones causing symptoms that are most often associated with menopause. This transition can last anywhere from a few months to a few years. As women learn more about hormones, they realize that they do not need to struggle with menopausal symptoms nor do they need to accept the physiological consequences of long-term deficiencies.

While hormone balancing may be straightforward for some women, for others it involves a dynamic process that requires a lot of fine-tuning. In this chapter, we'll take a look at the symptoms caused by less-than-optimal hormone levels of estrogen, progesterone and testosterone as well as the current options available to find relief.

WHAT IS HAPPENING TO MY BODY?

For decades, the symptoms of pre- and perimenopause were believed to be caused by a decline in estrogen. It is now understood that there is more to the story than just a decline in estrogen. In fact, hot flashes, the most famous symptom of menopause, are caused by fluctuations in both estrogen and progesterone. It is also known that fluctuations in testosterone can cause hot flashes, since testosterone can be converted into both estrogen and progesterone. Flashes can also be caused by other factors, such as a change in diet or stress level, which indirectly cause changes in hormone levels. The most important thing to understand about hot flashes is that they are caused by a *fluctuation* in hormone levels, which means that they often occur when you make adjustment in HRT levels.

Today, much more is known about symptoms that present themselves when there is a decline in ovarian hormones, and there is also more known about the symptoms that occur when hormone levels are *too high*. Let's look at the symptoms associated with deficiencies and excesses in all of the major female hormones:

Symptoms of Low Estrogen

Estrogens have significant effects on many parts of the body. Noticeable effects of low estrogen can include the following:

Dryness and loss of tissue elasticity
Loss of estrogen causes fragility and dryness in the tissues of the vagina and urinary tract.

Skin changes
A drop in estrogen levels results in noticeably thinner skin with less collagen and moisture.

Weakening of the genitourinary tract
Decreased estrogen levels can cause vaginal atrophy as well as a weakness in the muscles supporting the bladder, which may result in incontinence.

Cardiovascular changes
Because estrogen acts to lower blood pressure and relax arterial walls, a less-than-adequate supply may increase the risk of heart attacks.

Gum inflammation
Lowered estrogen levels cause destruction in the fibers of gum tissue.

Vision changes
Loss of estrogen also affects vision. For example, changes in eye shape may require corrections to eyeglasses and the fit of contacts, and dryness can lead to difficulty in wearing contacts.

Cholesterol levels
A decrease in estrogen causes an increase in LDL cholesterol (bad cholesterol) and a decrease in HDL cholesterol (good cholesterol), which may increase risk for heart disease.

Impact on the brain
Lowered estrogen causes depression and memory problems. Dr. Edward Klaiber, who wrote *Hormones and the Mind,* discovered a connection between estrogen and brain function accidentally in the 1970s while he was working with a colleague Dr. Yutaka Kobayashi, a biochemist at the Worcester Foundation. Kobayashi discovered an inverse relationship between a brain chemical called monoamine oxidase (MAO) and estrogen and testosterone. MAO breaks down norepinephine and serotonin, two major neurotransmitters that influence mood. When there is too little estrogen, there is too much MAO. This results in insufficient levels of norepinephine and serotonin, which is associated with depression and cognitive difficulties.

Bone density
A decrease in estrogen causes a loss of bone density and may eventually lead to osteoporosis.

Testosterone dominance
A drop in estrogen levels may cause a relative testosterone dominance

(because estrogen controls testosterone). Testosterone dominance can lead to female pattern hair loss and an impaired glucose metabolism.

Symptoms of High Estrogen

High levels of estrogen can be devastating to a woman's health. For example, the most well-known symptom is an over stimulation of the uterine lining (endometrium), which is listed below with other serious effects of high estrogen.

Stimulation of the endometrium
Estrogen's effect on cell multiplication causes a dangerous situation when this hormone is not opposed by progesterone. Estrogen's stimulation of the endometrium, or uterine lining, has been proven to cause cancer. In women who have endometriosis, this stimulating effect causes growth in bits of the endometrium, which can spread throughout the abdominal cavity.

Low thyroid
Excess estrogen binds or limits thyroid hormone. Symptoms of the subsequent low thyroid level include fatigue; forgetfulness; depression; cold intolerance; constipation; night blindness; hearing loss; weight gain; elevated cholesterol, hair, skin, and nail problems; heavy or more frequent menstrual cycles; snoring or sleep apnea, and aches in joints.

Suppression of orgasms
High levels of estrogen can dampen the intensity of an orgasm or prevent orgasm from occurring.

Symptoms of Low Progesterone

Because progesterone acts to oppose estrogen, the symptoms of low progesterone can look like the symptoms of high estrogen. This has led many practitioners to evaluate progesterone to estrogen in a P:E ratio. When the amount of progesterone is divided by the amount of estradiol, the resulting ratio can be correlated to symptoms. Dr. Joseph Collins, author of *What's Your Menopause Type?*, explains that your body should have between 20 to 170 molecules of progesterone to one molecule of estrogen. Values that are less than or greater than this range can cause health problems. A very low P:E ratio (too much estrogen relative to progesterone) can cause the following:

Irritability

Estrogen's excitatory effects can cause irritability, insomnia and anxiety.

Low thyroid

If estrogen binds or limits thyroid hormone, low progesterone means estrogen is suppressing the thyroid. Progesterone aids thyroid function by allowing for the retention of zinc and potassium in cells. These two elements allow thyroid hormone to enter a cell to be converted to T3, an active form of the hormone.

Pain and inflammation

Low progesterone can cause muscle aches and joint pains.

Excess growth in the uterine lining

Growth in the uterine lining is the result of unopposed estrogen indicating that there may not be enough progesterone.

Uterine bleeding

Uterine bleeding or spotting can be caused by a low P:E ratio, the result of low progesterone.

Hypoglycemia, allergies, and arthritis

Because progesterone is the major precursor of the important corticosteroid hormones (aldosterone and cortisol) made in the adrenal cortex, low progesterone can lead to hypoglycemia, allergies, and arthritis caused by problems with the body's mineral balance.

Symptoms of High Progesterone

A high P:E ratio (too much progesterone relative to estrogen) can cause the following:

Fatigue or drowsiness
Progesterone has a Valium-like effect on the nervous system which can cause drowsiness.

Bloating
Bloating is a symptom associated with synthetic progesterone.

Constipation
Progesterone is known to relax your gastrointestinal muscles and can slow down your bowel movements.

Insulin resistance
High progesterone levels similar to those observed in late pregnancy can induce a state of insulin resistance. Insulin is a hormone that builds body fat, and progesterone is an insulin trigger that promotes fat storage to provide fuel for a growing baby.

In pregnant women and women who have a hormone imbalance, increased body fat can cause insulin to be less efficient. Normally, insulin functions to move glucose out of the bloodstream—either to muscle or to fat for storage.

When insulin becomes less efficient or when insulin receptors become less responsive, blood glucose levels grow higher after eating, which causes even more insulin to be released. Sudden rushes of insulin after meals cause a reactive hypoglycemia response, causing hunger, shakiness and light-headedness. Unwise responses to food cravings for sweets cause this cycle to repeat itself over and over.

Symptoms of Low Testosterone

Although women's bodies make tiny amounts of testosterone each day (men produce 10 to 15 times more testosterone than women), we now know that symptoms of low testosterone in women include the following:

Lowered libido

Low levels of testosterone cause a diminished interest in sex as well as a decreased sensitivity to stimulation and lowered strength of orgasm. In *Hormone of Desire*, Dr. Susan Rako explains that there are testosterone receptors in a woman's nipples as well as in the clitoris and the vagina. When these receptors respond to available testosterone, it forms the basis for sexual pleasure.

Increased fat storage

Fat cells have both beta-receptors and alpha-receptors. Beta-receptors function to accelerate the release of fat, and alpha-receptors slow down the release of fat. Testosterone acts to increase the number of beta-receptors.

Increased irritability

Just as there are testosterone receptors in a woman's genitals, there are also testosterone receptors in the brain that contribute to a sense of well being. Lowered levels of testosterone can have a negative effect on a woman's mood.

Symptoms of High Testosterone

Testosterone is an anabolic hormone that builds protein. Too much can cause serious health problems. As a result, testosterone supplementation should be approached very cautiously. Excess testosterone can cause the following:

Elevated cholesterol

High testosterone has been shown to increase LDL cholesterol (bad cholesterol) and reduce HDL cholesterol (good cholesterol).

Increased virilization

Virilization refers to an increase in male characteristics—a deepening of the voice, increased body hair, acne, and an enlargement of the clitoris.

Aggressive behavior

High testosterone has been associated with aggressive behavior that includes anger, frustration and impatience.

SHOULD I HAVE A HORMONE TEST?

So many health practitioners and organizations are recommending hormone level testing because it seems like a wonderful tool. However, hormone balancing is difficult to accomplish with lab tests for a number of reasons:

- Hormone levels fluctuate a great deal, especially in pre- and perimenopause. Because of the cyclic nature of hormone levels and the complexities of hormone systems, hormone test result ranges are always quite wide. Women's "normal" ranges tend to vary a great deal, and reference points turn out to be very confusing.

- Blood tests cannot determine free estrogen or the amount that is available in your body. Instead, blood tests measure total serum estrogen, a value that is not very useful when trying to evaluate bio-available levels.

- Saliva tests for progesterone and estrogen give unreliable results because of hourly fluctuations. Also, saliva test results are abnormally high for women who use progesterone cream. This defeats the purpose of hormone testing once you have started hormone replacement therapy because it makes it impossible to test progesterone accurately.

Is Hormone Testing Ever a Good Idea?

If you have an extremely low or high level of hormones, tests can help you and your doctor correlate your symptoms. Although most women don't have test results at extreme levels, in these situations, the lab results are clearer and may give you peace of mind when you know your detective work is definitive.

WHAT HORMONES SHOULD I TAKE?

Hormone balancing is a process that may take several months of fine-tuning. In addition, there are many forms of hormone replacement therapy as well as dosages and delivery schedules. In this section, we'll start by looking at two categories of hormones:

- Bio-identical
- Synthetic

Bioidentical or Human-identical Hormones

Bio-identical refers to the molecular structure of hormones that are produced from plants. Although synthesized in a laboratory, the body sees a bio-identical hormone as *identical* to the hormones made in the body. These natural hormones are synthesized from fats extracted from wild yams or soybeans and are mostly available by prescription.

Synthetic or Patentable Hormones

Synthetic or patentable hormones are *not identical* to your body's own hormones. They are hormone molecules that are synthesized in the laboratory and altered slightly so they can be patented. Synthetic hormones are more widely marketed than bioidentical hormones because of the marketing efforts of large pharmaceutical companies. In contrast, most bio-identical hormones are made by a handful of compounding pharmacies that have existed since the early 1980s. Most medical doctors will only be familiar with synthetic hormones mentioned in textbooks on gynecology and obstetrics. While synthetic hormones have a reputation for causing more side effects than bio-identical hormones, some women have uncomfortable side effects when they take bio-identical hormones and prefer synthetics. Also, during pre- and perimenopause, many women use oral or transdermal contraceptives effectively to control symptoms. It's always up to a woman and her doctor to choose what's best for her.

DO I BALANCE MY HORMONES ALL AT ONCE?

Your doctor will want to evaluate your need for all of the major hormones. For example, women who have had a hysterectomy may be given estrogen alone so that there's only one variable when it comes to adjusting the dose. Sometimes progesterone will be added when symptoms of estrogen excess present themselves. Once progesterone is added, there will be two variables involved in fine-tuning with a need to decide whether to adjust one or both and in which direction.

Women in premenopause who have not had a hysterectomy will need to cycle estrogen and progesterone on a monthly basis to prevent endometrial cancer caused by unopposed estrogen. By peri-and postmenopause, cycling is usually not necessary, and continuous or daily dosing is often preferred. The conservative approach to adding testosterone would be to balance estrogen with progesterone before attempting to add testosterone. Because progesterone is a building block in the production of testosterone (see: Chapter 2, Figure 2), it is considered safer to see if the combination of estrogen and progesterone can generate adequate levels of testosterone in order to avoid the serious side effects of taking testosterone as a separate hormone.

Numerous other issues will need to be considered when starting hormone replacement therapy including the following:

Age

Younger women can require higher doses of hormones than older women.

Endometriosis

Because estrogen stimulates endometriosis tissue, the presence of this disease will require special attention because progesterone may need to be used to inhibit this growth. Some doctors like to prescribe progesterone by itself to shrink endometriosis tissue.

Thyroid Hormone Problems

Because of the interrelationships that exist between the thyroid system and ovarian hormones (see: "Symptoms of Low Estrogen and Symptoms of High Progesterone" in this chapter), women with thyroid problems may have a difficult time balancing their ovarian hormones. As a result, it is a good idea to treat a thyroid problem first.

Polycystic Ovarian Syndrome (PCOS)

This complex endocrine disorder which is characterized by high androgen levels, insulin resistance, and infertility, requires balancing of several hormone systems at once.

Alcohol

Because alcohol magnifies circulating estrogen levels, women who drink alcohol may require lower doses.

Tobacco

Tobacco counteracts the effect of estrogen. For women who smoke, increasing estrogen is not an option because of the risk of blood clots. Women who smoke who are considering HRT are advised to stop smoking, but smoking is not an absolute contraindication to HRT.

Stress

Stress influences the level of available progesterone in our bodies because progesterone is used as a precursor in cortisol production. Cortisol is the fight-or-flight stress hormone that is produced in the adrenal glands using progesterone as a building block. As a result, women who are coping with stress in their lives may need higher doses of progesterone.

WHAT FORMS OF HORMONES ARE AVAILABLE?

The forms of hormone replacement therapy are known as delivery systems. Choices include pills, patches, creams, shots, pellets, and vaginal rings. The hormonal benefits of various forms will vary from woman to woman. As result, part of hormone balancing involves finding a form that is best suited to your metabolic needs.

Oral Delivery Systems

Hormone pills are dissolved in the stomach and hormones are transported by the blood to the liver, where the hormone is processed. Although oral estrogens have a beneficial effect on cholesterol and blood lipids in *some women,* in other women, oral estrogen causes an increase in triglycerides, which is a risk factor for heart disease and diabetes. Pills are thought to be linked to fluid retention, and they also metabolize into high levels of estrone, which is a risk factor for breast cancer. As for dosing, pills can only be adjusted in multiples of pills. However, many women do very well on oral formulations, and sublingual under-the-tongue forms are also available.

Estrogens
The estrogens listed below all require a prescription. Oral synthetics are purchased from conventional pharmacies and most oral bio-identicals are purchased from compounding pharmacies with exceptions noted (see: "What is a Compounding Pharmacy?" in this chapter).

Oral Synthetics	Oral Bio-identicals
Cenestin	Biestrogen (Bi-Est)
Estratab	Estrace[*]
Femhrt	Triestrogen (Tri-Est), available in capsules, drops, suspension, or lozenges
Menest	
Ogen	
Ortho-Est	
Premarin	

    *   Available from a conventional pharmacy

Progesterone

Similar to estrogens, oral progesterones require a prescription, and the sources are the same: oral synthetics are purchased from conventional pharmacies, and most oral bio-identicals are purchased from compounding pharmacies with the noted exceptions.

Oral Progestins (Synthetics)	Oral Progesterone(Bio-identicals)
Aygestin	Prometrium[*]
Cycrin	Custom-compounded capsules, drops, suspension, or lozenges
Megace	
Micronor	
Nor-QD	
Provera	

    *   Available from a conventional pharmacy

Combination Estrogen and Progesterone

The following combination pills are considered convenient. A single product also costs less. However, the combined pill format prevents an individual adjustment of hormone doses.

Oral Synthetics	Oral Bio-identical
Activella	Custom-compounded capsules, drops, suspension, or lozenges
Femhrt	
Ortho-prefest	
Premphase	
Prempro	
Oral contraceptives	

Testosterone

Similar to estrogens, oral testosterone requires a prescription and the sources are the same: oral synthetics are purchased from conventional pharmacies, and oral bio-identicals are purchased from compounding pharmacies.

Oral Combo—Estrogen and Testosterone (Synthetic)	Oral Bio-identical
Estratest	Custom-compounded capsules
Menogen	

Transdermal Hormones

Transdermal hormones in the form of creams, gels, and patches are applied to the external skin. The hormones accumulate in layers of body fat and are released into the blood over time. In some women, this can lead to symptoms of excess. However, in general, hormones delivered by this method are

- not processed by the liver (first pass effect)

- preferable for women with clotting problems or liver disease

- often a better choice for women with high blood pressure

Although dosage levels of creams and gels are easier to adjust than pills, patches are somewhat challenging to adjust. Patch dosages may be adjusted by wearing two patches or possibly reduced by trimming.

Estrogens
The estrogens listed below all require prescriptions.

Cream/Gel Synthetics	Patch Bio-identicals[*]	Cream/Gel Bio-identicals
Estrasorb	Alora	Custom-compounded estrogens
	Climara	
	Esclim	
	Estraderm	
	Vivelle	
	Vivelle Dot	

* These bio-identicals contain only estradiol.

Progesterone
The progesterones listed below all require prescriptions.

Transdermal Progesterone (Bioidenticals)
Custom-compounded cream
Prochieve

Combination Estrogen and Progesterone

Like combination pills, the following patch and cream products are convenient to use.

Patch Synthetic	Transdermal Bio-identical
CombiPatch Ortho Evra Patch Contraceptive	Custom-compounded cream

Testosterone

Similar to estrogens, oral testosterone also requires a prescription.

Transdermal Synthetic	Transdermal Bio-identical
Methyltestosterone	Custom-compounded gel

Vaginal Hormones or Rectal Hormones

Vaginal or rectal hormones deliver hormones through mucous membranes. Delivery includes creams, gels, rings, suppositories, drops, and suspensions. Most of these are considered not systemically absorbed but can be, depending on the dose and system used.

Estrogens

The estrogens listed below all require a prescription.

Vaginal Synthetics	Vaginal Bio-identicals[*]
Premarin cream Femring (Menoring)	Vagifem Estring Estrace cream Custom-compounded forms[**]

[*] These bioidenticals contain only estradiol.
[**] These can also be used rectally.

Progesterone
The progesterones listed below all require prescriptions.

Vaginal Synthetics	Vaginal and Rectal Bio-identicals
Not used for hormone therapy	Custom-compounded forms

Testosterone
The estrogens listed below all require prescriptions.

Vaginal Synthetics	Vaginal and Rectal Bio-identicals
Not used for hormone therapy	Custom-compounded forms

Subdermal Hormones

Shots, pellets, and certain injections are considered to be subdermal hormones. These mechanisms are designed to be very slowly time released, extending over a period of one to three months.

Estrogens
The estrogens listed below all require administration by a health-care provider.

Subdermal Synthetics	Subdermal Bio-identicals
No subdermal synthetics exist	Delestrogen (estradiol valerate injection)

Progestin and Progesterone
The progestin and progesterone listed below require administration by a health-care provider.

Subdermal Synthetics	Subdermal Bio-identicals
Depo-provera	Custom-compounded forms
Contraceptive Implants	

Combination Estrogen and Progesterone

Like combination pills and creams, the following injectible product is considered convenient by some women.

Subdermal Synthetics
Lunelle Contraceptive Injection

Testosterone

Subdermal forms are not used for hormone replacement in women.

Intrauterine Hormones

An IUD containing levonorgestrel, a synthetic progestin, delivers this hormone 24 hours a day for 5 years. This is helpful to control bleeding in some women.

WHAT IS A COMPOUNDING PHARMACY?

Compounding pharmacies are small private pharmacies that prepare hormones for patients to a doctor's prescription specifications in pills, creams, gels, pellets, and implants. At one time, all pharmacists were compounding pharmacists.

Although compounding pharmacies are the only sources for prescription natural hormones, this valuable resource was almost eliminated. In 1997, President Bill Clinton signed the FDA Modernization Act, which prevented compounding pharmacies from advertising or marketing. That year, seven compounding pharmacies joined forces, sued the Food and Drug Administration and won in the U.S. Court of Appeals for the Ninth Circuit on the basis of freedom of speech. In 2002, the FDA took the case to the Supreme Court, where five of the nine Supreme Court justices voted in favor of the compounding pharmacies, representing a narrow but important victory.

All compounding pharmacies sell products by mail order by prescription. If you are not presently seeing a doctor who is familiar with natural hormones, compounding pharmacists can also help you locate a doctor in your area. In alphabetical order, the following list includes compounding pharmacies from around the United States:

Abrams Royal Pharmacy
8220 Abrams Road
Dallas, TX 75231
(214) 349-8000

California Pharmacy & Compounding Center
307 Placentia Aveue, Suite 102
Newport Beach, CA 92663
(800) 575-7776
(949) 642-8057
(714) 642-0725 (Fax)
www.californiapharmacy.com

College Pharmacy
833 North Tejon Street
Colorado Springs, CO 80903
(800) 888-9358
(719) 262-0022
(800) 556-5893
(719) 262-0035 (Fax)
E-mail: info@collegepharmacy.com
www.collegepharmacy.com

Hazle Drugs Apothecary Inc.
20 North Laurel Street
Hazleton, PA 18201
(570) 454-2670
(800) 439-2026
(800) 400-8764 (Fax)
E-mail: info@hazledrugs.com
www.hazledrugs.com

Hopewell Pharmacy and Compounding Center
One West Broad Street
Hopewell, NJ 08525
(609) 466-1960
(800) 792-6670
(800) 417-3864
info@hopewellrx.com
www.hopewellrx.com

Kronos Science Laboratory
3675 South Rainbow Boulevard, Suite 103
Las Vegas, Nevada 89103
(800) 723-7455
(702) 873-8455
(702) 873-6845 (Fax)
E-mail: info@kronospharmacy.com
www.KronosPharmacy.com

Lakeside Pharmacy
4632 Highway 58 North
Chattanooga, TN 37416
(423) 894-3222
(800) 523-1486
(423) 499-8435 (Fax)
info@lakesidepharmacy.com
info@lakesidepharmacy.com

Madison Pharmacy Associates, Inc.
Women's Health America Group
1289 Deming Way
Madison, WI 53717
(800) 558-7046
(888) 898-7412 (Fax)

wha@womenshealth.com
www.womenshealth.com

Monument Pharmacy
115C Second Street, P.O. Box 511
Monument, CO 80132
(719) 481-2209
(800) 595-7565
(719) 481-4971 (Fax)
E-mail: monpharm@rmi.net
www.monumentpharmacy.com

Wellness Health & Pharmaceutical
2800 South Eighteenth Street
Birmingham, AL 35209
(205) 879-6551
(800) 227-2627
(205) 871-2568 (Fax)
(800) 369-0302 (Fax)

Women's International Pharmacy
5708 Monona Drive
Madison, WI 53716-3152
(608) 221-7800
(800) 699-8144
(608) 221-7819 (Fax)
(800) 613-8862 (Fax)
www.womensinternational.com

Women's International Pharmacy
12012 North 111th Avenue
Youngtown, AZ 85363
(623) 214-7700
(800) 699-8143

(623) 214-7708 (Fax)
(800) 330-0268 (Fax)
www.womensinternational.com

To find additional listings of compounding pharmacists in the United States, Canada, Australia, and New Zealand, contact the following:

International Academy of Compounding Pharmacists (IACP)
P.O. Box 1365
Sugar Land, TX 77487
(281) 933-8400
(800) 927-4227
http://www.iacprx.org

Professional Compounding Centers of America (PCCA)
9901 South Wilcrest Drive
Houston, TX 77099
(800) 331-2498
(281) 933-6948
http://www.pccarx.com

Choosing Your Hormones

It's advisable to work with your doctor to choose the form and dosage of HRT that is right for you. Your physician's knowledge about what is available will help you make your decision. Remember that your doctor's experience with various formulations is invaluable. Remember too that your decision is not cast in stone. You can try different forms and doses over time. A trial period of three months with any of the above forms will provide an opportunity to gauge your needs. You can try the alternatives until your goals are met.

Establish a Ritual to Remember to Take Your Hormones

If you start taking hormone pills or cream, you will need to establish a daily reminder to take the hormones. Patches will require that you establish either a once-a-week or twice-a-week ritual to change your patch. Keeping your body supplied with a steady, consistent supply of supplemental hormones will prevent the wobble or fluctuation associated with hot flashes so it's important to remember to take your hormones consistently.

The Estrogenic Effect of Food and Herbs

Foods and herbs that have an estrogenic effect on the body can be so potent that some health practitioners see them as an alternative to hormone replacement therapy. For women who cannot take hormones, this may be a good thing, but for women who are carefully planning an HRT strategy, the wrong foods and herbs can disrupt the balance they're trying hard to achieve. For details concerning the hormone properties of foods and herbs, see Chapter 6.

Chart Your Symptoms

Charting your symptoms can be useful when you begin hormone replacement therapy because it provides a history of when the symptoms occurred.

A chart that helps you track symptoms as you begin hormone replacement therapy—similar to the Premenopause and Perimenopause symptom chart presented in the previous chapter—will help you track symptoms as your begin hormone replacement therapy. The chart will help you communicate with your doctor and relay exactly what is happening in your body.

HRT Symptom Chart

Month Day			
1			
2			
3			
4			
5			
6			
7			
8			
9			
10			
11			
12			
13			
14			
15			
16			
17			
18			
19			
20			
21			
22			
23			
24			
25			
26			
27			
28			
29			
30			
31			

Figure 6.

Steps for Completing the Chart:

1. Either enlarge the chart on the previous page with a photocopier or use it as a guide to create your own.

   Depending on how you feel about a larger form, you might consider using a blank book or a dated journal. A larger journal will give you an opportunity to include notes about your emotional changes, the food you eat, your exercise, and the stress you experience.

2. If you do use the chart provided, notice that the numbers in the left column of the chart correspond to the days of the month. Use the space at the top of each column to label the months you are charting. Because you may want to chart your symptoms for several months, you may want to add the year.

3. Use the following chart as a guide for charting:

Letter	Symptom
X	Took Your Hormones
F	Flash (Hot Flash)
S	Sweat (Night Sweat)
B	Breast tenderness
H	Headaches
C	Cramps
WR	Water Retention
I	Irritability
L	Lethargy

6.   (Option) Use the following numbers to chart the severity of your symptoms:

Number	Severity
1	Mild
2	Moderate
3	Severe

Support Groups

Ever since the sixties and seventies, women have been forming support groups to network and vent their feelings. Groups can be beneficial in helping women explore emotional issues surrounding menopause.

Since 1995, the Internet has provided many virtual support groups that bring people together from around the world. Examples include these two:

iVillage.com
iVillage.com is a women's portal that hosts thousands of message boards including a board on menopause and perimenopause.
http://messageboards.ivillage.com

webmd.com
WebMD is a health portal with message boards for hundreds of support groups including the following:

- Menopause

- Endometriosis

- PCOS

- Thyroid Disorders

- Bone Health: Density and Osteoporosis

http://boards.health.msn.com/roundtable.asp

Baseline Bone Screening

In the United States today, 10 million individuals already have osteoporosis and 18 million more have low bone mass, placing them at increased risk for osteoporosis. Numerous factors can be used to predict osteoporosis including the following:

Irregular periods

A menstrual period that deviates from your average cycle length and timing is considered to be irregular. Menstrual problems in adolescence or early adulthood can point to problems in bone development. Women attain 40 percent of bone mass during the first 20 years of life. This bone mass forms the foundation for bone resorption and remodeling for the rest of a woman's life. Early bone development is considered to be 80 percent related to genetic factors and 20 percent influenced by environmental factors such as nutrition, athletic training and calcium intake.

When a young female athlete restricts the amount or types of food she eats, she will indirectly cause changes in estrogen production in her body. Hundreds of calories are burned through exercise, and to conserve energy, the body will decrease or stop ovulating. This results in a drop in estrogen and skipped periods. Without sufficient estrogen and nutrition, bone development slows and bone loss may even occur.

Small Frame

Caucasian and Asian women are more prone to osteoporosis than African-American women.

Low dietary calcium

Poor dietary nutrition in adolescence related to heavy athletic activity, dieting, and eating disorders like anorexia and bulimia can lead to low calcium intake and low bone mass. High quantities of soda that is high in phosphates also interferes with calcium absorption.

Perimenopausal women should consider getting a baseline bone density screening test. Baseline screening provides a snapshot of bone density before estrogen levels decline and provides a valuable reference for screening later in life.

In perimenopausal women, the amount of bone density measured will be compared with an average measurement found in healthy young womens and the result will be expressed as a "T score." If a T score is positive, a woman's bone density is higher than that of a 30 year-old woman. A negative score represents a bone density that is less than that of a 30 year-old woman.

Types of bone density tests include the following:

Central DXA

The central dual X-ray absorptiometry machine is considered to be the best device for measuring bone density. Bone density is best evaluated at the spine and hip. This test usually takes five or ten minutes.

Ultrasound

Ultrasound devices are portable and can measure bone in the heel and forearm. Although this device is considered less precise than the central DXA, experts feel some measurement of bone density is better than no measurement. Because ultrasound devices are approximately the size of a laser printer, they have become popular screening devices at health fairs and shopping malls. If bone loss is noted on an ultrasound, then a full densitometer by DXA is recommended.

Diet and Supplements

Healthful nutrition positively affects hormone function throughout a woman's life, and it also helps maintain bone mass. Although menopause is an inevitable part of aging, many problems can be avoided by giving your body what it needs.

PART III

▼

STAYING HEALTHY AT THIS STAGE IN YOUR LIFE

Although women's hormone health has benefited from HRT, the wisdom of monitoring and maintaining your health through diet and lifestyle factors should not be overlooked.

By becoming aware of all your health options, you will be able to deal effectively with any health issues that may arise.

Although much of this section covers issues that arise "after HRT," there are many details, tips, and ideas that are pertinent for women of all ages.

CHAPTER 5

▼

WHAT'S NEXT?

For women who understand the risks and benefits of staying on HRT, the option exists to stay on hormones long term, and some doctors feel that this is beneficial for many women. However, other doctors are now recommending five years as the maximum amount of time women should take hormones with a transition that is accomplished progressively by taking smaller and smaller doses. For many women, this transition will be symptom free, but for some it may bring on a return of the symptoms that first led them to take hormones. This group will need to rebalance through trial and error, dosing until symptoms subside, or they may choose to restart hormone therapy.

This chapter introduces options available to women if they choose to make the transition to lower doses of HRT after menopause and includes the following:

- Super low dosing

- Tapering off hormones completely

- Low dose vaginal rings

- The truth about botanicals

SUPER LOW DOSING AFTER MENOPAUSE

As discusses in Part 2, older women require lower doses of hormones than younger women. As you get older, you may need to taper off your hormone dosages as your body's requirements change. If you're interested in tapering your dosages to go off hormones completely, you'll need to work with your doctor to plan lower doses on an appropriate timetable. Although there is no medical reason why you can't stop hormones cold turkey, an abrupt change in hormone levels increases the likelihood of symptoms. Experience has shown that it is best to give yourself at least a year to taper off hormones gradually.

How to Taper Off

Whether you're using oral hormones, a cream, or a patch, you'll want to plan a method to slowly decrease your dose. Here are some examples:

Oral Formulas

Try a gradual transition from one hormone tablet a day to one every other day for one month, and log your symptoms in a journal. If this is successful and you're symptom free, take one hormone tablet twice a week for four weeks followed by one tablet a week the following month. If you do not experience any severe symptoms, you will have successfully made the transition.

Transdermal Formulas

The formula in patches can be tapered slowly by cutting off small amounts of the patch. Dr. Michael Goodman, who wrote *The Midlife Bible*, recommends tapering very slowly by cutting off 10 to 20 percent of the patch one month at a time.

What to Expect

Just as it took time for your body to adjust to extra hormones when you started HRT, it may take time for your body to adjust to lower dosing. Some women experience no symptoms but others may experience hot flashes that we've said reflect the wobble of changing hormone levels. Although some women have gone off hormones abruptly without symptoms, every woman's body is different. Some experience a return of symptoms and then find that they need to go back on hormones and try to taper off months later.

CARDIAC HEALTH AFTER HRT

Be sure to ask your doctor to monitor lipid panels (a complete cholesterol panel) to assess the effect of HRT compared to no HRT. Some women's cholesterol panels become much more risky after stopping HRT. Some women may need medication and adjustments in their diet. A stress test with a scan is also frequently used to monitor cardiac health at any age.

BONE HEALTH AFTER HRT

Once you're off hormones, it is important to ask your doctor to monitor your bone health, make sure your vitamin and mineral intake is adequate, and create a strategy to add strength training to your weekly regimen.

Nutritional Supplements

Of the nutritional supplements mentioned in Chapter 6 (see: "Preventing Osteoporosis"), Vitamin K is the nutrient that is often overlooked, yet is critically important for bone health. Although it is mostly known for its role in blood clot formation, it is also required for the synthesis of osteocalcin, a protein produced by osteoblast cells, which build bone. Dr. Joseph Mercola, author of *The No Grain Diet* calls Vitamin K "glue that helps plug calcium into your bone matrix." (Note: women who take blood-thinning medications such as Coumadin, Heparin, and other related compounds should not take Vitamin K).

Strength Training

As you use the muscles of your body during weight bearing exercise, pressure is applied to your bones that results in a small amount of new bone formation. At the Jean Mayer Human Nutrition Research Center on Aging (of the U.S. Department of Agriculture—USDA) at Boston's Tufts University, researchers examined 39 sedentary women between the ages of 50 and 70. Twenty of the women who started a strength-training program gained 1 percent in bone density after a year and the sedentary group lost 2.5 percent.

Dr. Miriam E. Nelson, who is associate chief of the Human Physiology Laboratory at the center and author of *Strong Women Stay Young*, says that in our early forties, we start to lose about 1 percent of our muscle mass every year.

> *When we lose muscle, our metabolism drops, we don't have as much energy, we have problems with glucose intolerance, bone density drops, a whole host of sort of age-related chronic conditions happen. What we see with the strength training is that even over a couple of decades, the research is showing us that people don't lose any muscle when they're lifting weights just two or three times a week.*

Muscles in the upper and lower body can be strengthened with strength-training equipment at a gym or at home with free weights. If you don't own weights, household items such as soup cans may be used. Start by lifting a weight you can lift without very much effort 5 times. When this becomes too easy, increase repetitions to 2 sets of 5, and then 3 sets of 5. Move up to 10 repetitions in each set, and then increase to 15 times in each set. When this becomes easy, increase the weight you are lifting. Try to do strength-training exercises for 30–40 minutes 2–3 times a week.

In some cases prescription medications such as Fosamax or Actonel are used to stop bone loss and sometimes even reverse it. Taking a medication of this type is an important subject to discuss with your doctor.

SKIN HEALTH AFTER HRT

Women of all ages are aware of simple measures for taking care of their skin. These include keeping the skin moisturized and wearing sun block when outdoors. This section contains a few lesser-known nutritional therapies.

Vitamin K and C

In his book *What's Your Menopause Type?*, Dr. Joseph Collins describes animal studies that have helped researchers make a connection between vitamin K and the thinning skin that occurs at menopause. Research has shown that a vitamin K deficiency can cause an increased breakdown in skin collagen and a decrease in the total amount of skin collagen. Collins also explains that a synergy exists between vitamin K and vitamin C that is not fully understood. For example, scientists recognize a deficiency of vitamin K associated with a drop in vitamin C levels in the adrenal glands, liver and other tissues. Because vitamin K helps the blood to clot properly, the only women who would need to be concerned about vitamin K supplements are those who are taking blood-thinners. Otherwise, vitamin K may be taken in doses of up to 1,000 micrograms a day (1 milligram). Dr. Linus Pauling, who was the first to recognize the importance of vitamin C, recommended a daily intake of 1,000 milligrams or more.

Essential Fatty Acids

Udo Erasmus, who wrote *Fats That Heal Fats That Kill*, explains that oils rich in essential fatty acids (EFAs) nourish the skin, hair and nails. This subject may be one of the most complex topics in human nutrition but well worth exploring. Because EFAs are an important part of human nutrition, you may also want to spread the word to family members. Here are some important points:

Essential Fatty Acids Must Be Obtained from Food

Omega-6 (LA) and omega-3 (LNA) fatty acids are polyunsaturated fats that are called essential because we need to obtain them from food. In contrast, nonessential amino acids can be manufactured out of other chemicals found in your body.

Essential Fatty Acids Must Be Balanced

Omega-6 (LA) and omega-3 (LNA) fatty acids must be balanced for an optimum effect. These fatty acids compete for receptor sites in cell membranes, where they play a critical role in cellular function.

An optimum ratio of omega-6 (LA) to omega-3 (LNA) in the diet is between 2 to 1 and 5 to 1. In other words, the ideal ratio is 2 to 5 times as much omega-6 fatty acids as omega-3 fatty acids. Most Americans consume 10 or 15 times more omega-6 than omega-3 fatty acids, which means *omega-3 fatty acids need to be boosted*.

Flax is a Rich Source of Omega-3

Author Udo Erasmus explains that flaxseed oil, containing the richest plant-based source of omega-3 fatty acid, is a quick way to make up for a long-standing omega-3 deficiency. However, because flaxseed oil contains four times more omega-3s than omega-6s, its long-term use can result in omega-6 deficiency symptoms that can occur in 16 months to 2 years (see: "Deficiency Symptoms" later in this section). Manufacturers who understand this have been producing oil blends.

Try to buy only cold-pressed, nonrefined oils, and store them in the refrigerator away from light and air. When flaxseed oil is purchased, it deteriorates unless it is refrigerated. It is also important to note that oxygen and light both contribute to rancidity of *all* oils. It makes sense, therefore, to buy oils in metal cans or opague bottles.

Fish Are a Rich Source of Omega-3 Fatty Acids

Fish, particularly sardines and salmon, have high levels of omega-3 fatty acids, but there are contaminants in fish that are worrisome. The Environmental Working Group found that farm-raised salmon has greater amounts of polychlorinated biphenyls, or PCBs, than wild salmon (PCBs are known carcinogens in animals and are a suspected one in humans).

It is important to note that long-chain Omega-3 essential fatty acids known as EPA and DHA are found most abundantly inside many cold water fish. Shorter-chain Omega-3s found in canola and flaxseed oil must be converted by the body to EPA and DHA to obtain the benefits of these oils.

EPA is a regulator of enzymes that control the conversion of the Omega-6 fatty acids.

DHA is critical for many cell membranes to transfer information and for the retina to receive visual input. Brain cells are also dependent on adequate levels of DHA.

Because fish oil contain EPA and DHA, and because fish are contaminated with organic mercury, PCBs, and DDT, many supplement manufacturers have started to offer pharmaceutical-grade, molecularly distilled fish oil supplements that are free of pollutants. Be sure to ask for a pharmaeutical-grade when you're shopping for fish oil supplements.

Grass-Fed Animals Contain Omega-3 Fatty Acids
Meats and milks from grass-fed animals are thought to be nutritionally superior to grain-fed animal products. Although grass-fed animals are often smaller and weigh less than grain-fattened animals, they contain less total fat, less saturated fat, less omega-6 fat, and far more vitamins, minerals, and beneficial fats, including omega-3 fats. Pasture-raised chickens produce meat and eggs high in vitamins, minerals, flavonoids, and omega-3 fatty acids, but they are low in undesirable omega-6 fatty acids. In contrast, chickens fed organic corn and soy meal are comparatively much lower in vitamins, minerals, flavonoids, and omega-3 fatty acids and much higher in omega-6 fatty acids.

Processed Foods and Omega-6 Oil
Most processed foods, such as breads, cookies, cakes, crackers, chips, doughnuts, muffins, cereals—and all fast foods—are made using

omega-6 vegetable oils. In addition, most of these foods are also made with hydrogenated fats which contain the harmful trans fats.

Oils Containing Both Omega-3 and Omega-6

Flax seed, hemp seed, and black current seed oils are nutritionally superior to other plant-based oils because they contain both omega-3 and omega-6 fatty acids. Notice the content of popular oils sold in health food stores as supplements:

Oil	Omega-6 (LA)	Omega-3 (LNA)
Flax Seed	15.2%	50.1%
Black Current Seed	47.1%	13.1%
Borage Seed	40.3%	N/A
Hemp Seed	55%	25%

Tips for Boosting Omega-3 Fatty Acids

When you flood your diet with omega-6 fatty acids, they compete against omega-3s for entry into key cells in the heart and brain. This makes it more difficult for your body and brain to get enough omega-3s. Here are some tips for how to obtain enough omega-3 fatty acids:

- **Use olive oil**
  Although there's not a large amount of omega-3 in olive oil, it is better than corn, safflower, and soybean oil, all of which are high in omega-6 fatty acids.

- **Beware of oil in canned goods and processed food**
  Tuna and other products packed in cans often contain large amounts of soybean oil. Soybean oil's omega-6 content will overwhelm the omega-3s.

- **Avocados and nuts contain high levels of omega-6**
  The confusion over avocados and nuts indicates that the subject of EFAs is complex. Although avocados are often described as good sources of omega-3s, they have about 16

times as many omega-6s as omega-3s. Nuts provide omega-3 fatty acids, but also a lot of omega-6s. These foods would overwhelm your omega-3s.

Examples of fruits and vegetables that contain omega-3 fatty acids include wild rice, kidney beans, melon, spinach, cauliflower, broccoli, Boston lettuce, and cherries.

- **Omega-6 Fatty Acid (LA) Deficiency Symptoms**
  Essential fatty acids are necessary for the normal functioning of the reproductive system, hormone regulation, and for breaking up cholesterol deposits in the arteries. Deficiencies cause changes in cell structure that result in slowed growth. Omega-6 deficiency symptoms include

  ----

  Weakness

  Vision impairment

  Tingling (arms and legs)

  Motor incoordination

- **Omega-3 Fatty Acid (LNA) Deficiency Symptoms**
  Essential fatty acids are constituents of all cell membranes in all body tissues. They are also precursors to prostaglandins that influence immune, cardiovascular, secretory, digestive, and reproductive functions. Omega-3 deficiency symptoms include

  ----

  Dry, scaly skin

  Excessive thirst

Fatigue

Dandruff and/or hair loss

Frequent urination

Vision impairment

Impaired memory

Brittle or soft nails

Depression

BLADDER HEALTH AFTER HRT

It is estimated that 5 to15 percent of women aged 15 to 75 years suffer from urinary incontinence, but only 25 percent seek help. Menopause is not the only cause of poor bladder control. A similar muscle weakness is sometimes caused by childbirth. The most common types of urinary incontinence are stress and urge incontinence:

Stress Incontinence

Stress incontinence is the most common type (40 percent), and it occurs during a physical activity such as laughing, sneezing, coughing, lifting something heavy, or exercising. Pelvic floor muscle training has been shown to be very effective. In a Women's Hospital study at the University of Southern California School of Medicine, Los Angeles, 36 women with stress urinary incontinence were evaluated after three months of pelvic muscle exercises. Results showed that 20 patients (56 percent) were cured or substantially improved after completing the pelvic muscle training, whereas 16 were unchanged.

Kegel exercises are pelvic-muscle exercises named after Dr. Arnold Kegel, who developed a method of controlling incontinence in women following childbirth. In 1948, Kegel introduced regular daily exercising of pelvic muscles that improved urethral sphincter function.

In order to do Kegel exercises correctly, first experiment by locating the pelvic floor muscles that need to be exercised. This can be done while you are urinating by contracting the muscles that stop the urine flow. Contract these muscles repetitively until you become familiar with the contraction of this group of muscles. You should not contract your abdominal, thigh, or buttocks muscles while performing the exercise. Once you have identified the correct group of muscles, you can do Kegel exercises almost anywhere. You can, for example, exercise your pelvic floor muscles while you're driving a car, watching TV, or working at your desk. Try to hold a contraction for about 10 seconds and then rest the muscles for 10 seconds, doing a total of 10 contractions 3 or 4 times a day for at least 8 weeks. While some women may notice an improvement after a few weeks, others may not notice any change in bladder control for at least 6 to 12 weeks.

There are also simple surgical procedures that can relieve this problem. A pessary, a support that is inserted vaginally, can also be very helpful. Discuss these options with your doctor to see if one is right for you.

Urge Incontinence
Urge or reflex incontinence produces an overwhelming urge to urinate. Women with this type of incontinence experience difficulty getting to the bathroom in time. This type of incontinence is not caused by muscle weakness but by frequent bladder infections, nerve damage, diabetes, dementia, Alzheimer's, Parkinson's, and stroke. Treatment for this type of incontinence involves medication.

LOW-DOSE VAGINAL RINGS

Vaginal itching, dryness, painful intercourse, urinary urgency, and painful urination are symptoms of a condition known as urogenital atrophy (UGA). It is caused by long-term estrogen deficiency. Unlike hot flashes, these local vaginal and urinary symptoms of estrogen deficiency do not go away. Because symptoms of UGA often develop slowly, many women incorrectly assume these problems are part of aging. Fortunately, this condition may now be treated with a very low dose of estradiol through a small, flexible two-inch ring that is inserted into the vagina.

The estradiol in this product, called Estring, is delivered continuously over a 24-hour period for a total of 90 days. Made from yams, this bio-identical estrogen is delivered in extremely low doses to local tissues with very little effect on the rest of the body. Because there is little systemic exposure, the low dosing (6.5 to 9.5 micrograms) will not affect other symptoms of menopause.

Estring was first approved in Sweden in 1993 and is currently available in many countries, including the United Kingdom, Canada, New Zealand, South Africa, and Switzerland, as well as in the United States.

Vaginal estrogen creams also work in a similar way to alleviate urogenital atrophy (UGA).

THE TRUTH ABOUT BOTANICALS

Are botanical products (otherwise known as phytoestrogens) beneficial for women at menopause? At the present, only black cohosh seems to have gained widespread acceptance within the medical community. In 2001, the American College of Obstetricians and Gynecologists stated, "Black cohosh may be helpful in the short term (6 months or less) for women with vasomotor symptoms of menopause." (Note: Vasomotor refers to hot flashes and night sweats).

Natural May Not Mean Safe

Although herbs are gaining acceptance by the medical community, for the most part, little is known about their safety, potency, or chemical properties. Plant-based products sold in the supplement departments of health food stores are very accessible and they're beginning to occupy more and more space. Although it may be true that some phytoestrogens relieve the symptoms of menopause, herbs are potent medications and your decision to take them should be discussed with your doctor.

Without realizing it, many women may be self-medicating themselves with food products or supplements that have a hormone-like effect. In some cases, these products may be making their symptoms worse. For example, women who have had cancer or who are at risk for cancer, may be putting themselves in a dangerous situation by taking certain herbs that mimic estrogen. When herbs were tested at the University of Pittsburgh Cancer Institute, Dr. Patricia Eagon, associate professor of medicine, had this to say about the test results:

> *Our results indicate that some herbal remedies demonstrate measurable estrogenic activity, in spite of the fact that they are not traditionally used as such. This is important since it suggests that some extracts may not be appropriate for women who have a family or personal history of cancers that are linked to higher levels of estrogen, including breast and uterine cancer.*

Plant extracts were given to female rats whose ovaries had been removed to see whether the herbs would interact with the animals' estrogen receptors, as normal estrogen does. The researchers discovered the following reactions to various plants:

Herbs with a strong estrogen effect
Motherwort leaf
Saw palmetto berry
Rhodiola rosea root
Red clover blossom

Herbs with a moderate estrogen effect
Dong quai root
Black and blue cohosh
Vitex berry
Hops flower
Wild yam
Licorice root

Herbs with a weak estrogen effect
Maca root
Cramp bark
Turmeric root

Other Herbs, Other Studies

Sixty-eight million Americans now frequent health food stores, where food and supplement manufacturers have launched aggressive marketing campaigns aimed at menopausal women. This stampede has prompted research organizations to take a serious look at plant-based products.

As of this writing, the National Center for Complementary and Alternative Medicine (NCCAM) is recruiting patients (August 2003) for a study that will determine if black cohosh extract (BCE) results in estrogenic stimulation of the breast.

In a randomized, double-blind, placebo-controlled study to last twelve months commencing August 1, 2003, the National Institute of Aging (NIA) will compare the effects of three alternative treatments on menopausal symptoms using phytoestrogens, hormone replacement therapy, and placebo. The herbal formulas will contain black cohosh, alfalfa, chasteberry, dong quai, false unicorn, licorice, oats, pomegranate, siberian ginseng, and soy.

Soy Foods and Supplements

None of the phytoestrogen products that are marketed to menopausal women receive as much attention as soy. Health food stores and supermarkets are full of soy—burgers, hot dogs, cheeses, yogurt, milk, and ice cream, to name just a few. Soy derivatives are found in 60 to 70 percent of all processed food. Soy has also crept into food made for infants and pets. Marketers are promoting soy as a food that will reverse osteoporosis, ease the symptoms of menopause and PMS, reduce the risk of heart disease, and lower cholesterol.

With 140 billion pounds of soy produced in the United States each year, soy is big business. As a result, the soy industry's influence is very strong in the media, in research institutions, and in government agencies. Unfortunately, there is little mention of the following facts:

• Soy is one of the most heavily sprayed crops

• Soybeans have been subjected to genetic engineering (Note: New genetically engineered plants produce an insect toxin as they grow—in every cell of the plant throughout the entire growing season).

• There are chemicals in soy that can seriously harm your health

Because of the marketing dollars that are spent on soy, we hear more good news than bad news. Sometimes, however, the truth about soy's effects on health surfaces. In June of 2000, ABC's *20/20* aired a story on the dangers of soy when Daniel Doerge and Daniel Sheehan, both research scientists for the FDA and experts on soy, stepped forward to talk about the food's adverse effects. It turns out that the two scientists had signed a letter of protest to the FDA (their employer) because of their concern over studies showing a possible link between soy and breast cancer, diminished brain function in men, and developmental abnormalities in infants. The protest was in response to an FDA health claim concluding that soy may lower both cholesterol levels and the risk of heart disease.

In summary, more studies are needed to establish the benefits and risks of excess soy consumption.

CHAPTER 6

▼

PREVENTABLE DISEASE AT MENOPAUSE AND POSTMENOPAUSE

For many women, the symptoms associated with menopause will settle down when the body adapts to lower levels of hormone production. In the difficult years when hormones cause uncomfortable symptoms, hormone replacement therapy has been shown to be very effective in helping women past the "wobble."

Since the 1979s, pharmaceutical companies have been telling us that hormones protect women from the diseases of aging. Although it is true that a majority of women do not suffer from heart attacks or breast cancer in their twenties, when hormone levels are high, this does not mean that supplemental hormones will automatically protect women from degenerative disease, although it's possible they may. Further studies are needed in this area also.

HORMONES AND DISEASES OF AGING

Let's look at what's been said about the protective role of hormones when it comes to heart attacks, osteoporosis, and Alzheimer's disease and compare it to what we know:

Heart Disease

Although there have been several studies linking estrogen use to a reduction in heart disease, it is now known that hormones are not foolproof when it comes to preventing heart disease. Various studies have indicated that estrogen slows the development of atherosclerotic plaque, lowers cholesterol, increases blood flow, reduces the levels of a clotting factor called fibrinogen, and lowers blood pressure much as antihypertension medication does. In spite of these benefits, the truth is, as we get older, changes take place in the heart and the blood vessels that lead to deterioration in function. Flexibility in heart muscle walls decreases with age, ventricle walls thicken and become stiff, arteries stiffen because of changes in elastin and collagen, and valves begin to show signs of wear and tear. As we age, the risks for heart disease continue to rise, but hormones may slow that risk. The WHI study showed a small increase in cardiac events only in the first year of HRT. However, the study may have included many women who already had established heart disease.

Osteoporosis

As mentioned in Chapter 4 (see: "Baseline Bone Screening"), skeletal bone formation takes place before the age of 30. After the age of 30, the acquisition of bone mineral density stops and peak bone mass is maintained through a process known as remodeling. Remodeling is a hormone-controlled process that involves a continuous breakdown and reformation of small sections of bone. For women at menopause, the administration of estrogen prevents an increase in the rate of bone breakdown.

In the remodeling process, breakdown is called resorption and is performed by cells called osteoclasts. Bone-forming cells are called osteoblasts and fill in the holes created by resorption. A loss of bone density occurs as we age because osteoblasts are less efficient at *making* bone than the osteoclasts are at *removing* it.

At menopause, the loss of estrogen enhances the ability of osteoclasts to absorb bone. Since the osteoblasts cannot keep up by making new bone, more bone is lost than is produced. By reducing the rate at which remodeling occurs, estrogen supplementation prevents bone loss.

Alzheimer's Disease

In May of 2003, it was reported that the memory substudy of the Women's Health Initiative (WHI) found a heightened risk of developing dementia in a study of women 65 and older taking estrogen plus progestin hormone therapy. Again, these women were much older when hormones were started, so they may already have had established dementia. In his book, *Hormones and the Mind*, Dr. Edward Klaiber explains that in spite of several encouraging studies that have shown a reduction in Alzheimer's disease in women who use estrogen, there is no positive proof that estrogen protects the brain against Alzheimer's disease. He does point out that there is data to suggest that estrogen treatment can slow or reverse symptoms in at least some of the patients who already have Alzheimer's. However, he also says that there is data contradicting this suggestion.

Cancer

Cancer is thought to be caused by DNA mutations that are more likely to occur in older cells. Every time a cell divides, it is vulnerable to damage from mutation. Older cells have undergone many more divisions than younger cells. When death rates from cancer in women on HRT are compared with death rates from cancer in women not on HRT, the rates are very similar.

The proliferative effect of estrogen on cell multiplication has made estrogen a risk factor in tissues where normal cell division takes place in preparation for pregnancy: the ovaries, uterus, cervix (part of the uterus), and breast.

Although HRT *may* increase your risk of breast cancer, hormone replacement therapy protects against colon cancer. Compared with women who have never used HRT, women who have used hormones have a 20 percent lower incidence of colon cancer. While women are actually on HRT, there is a 30 percent lowering of colon cancer risk. It is thought that hormones *may* protect against colon cancer by helping to clear away bile salts, which are known to cause cancer.

Among the female hormones, progesterone has more of a reputation as a protector than estrogen. In the 1970s, estrogen was used alone to treat menopausal symptoms. When studies began to show that estrogen could lead to endometrial cancer, a progestin (synthetic progesterone) was added to estrogen therapy to protect the uterus. As an estrogen antagonist, progesterone prevents the buildup of excess tissue in the endometrium. Without progesterone, that formation can cause abnormally heavy flow during menstruation and spotting between periods. It may also lead to abnormal cells in the uterine lining.

Is Chronic Disease Preventable?

Although life expectancy statistics indicate that Americans live longer than their ancestors, statistics also show that we are heavier and more sedentary than ever before. In addition, the American health-care system, which emphasizes acute care over disease prevention, has trained Americans to *wait* for a magic pill.

Chronic diseases are considered to be the most preventable of all health problems, but prevention requires less passivity and more do-it-yourself changes. Because chronic disease originates in health-damaging behaviors, we will need to unlearn much of what we've been taught and start afresh with lifestyle changes, including the following:

Diet

In February 2002, the World Health Organization (WHO) hosted a conference on Diet, Nutrition and the Prevention of Chronic Diseases. The panel of experts at the conference concluded:

"Rapid changes in diets and lifestyles that have occurred with industrialization, urbanization, economic development and market globalization have accelerated over the past decade. While standards of living have improved in both developed and developing countries, there have been significant negative consequences in terms of inappropriate dietary patterns, decreased physical activities and a corresponding increase in diet-related chronic diseases. Examples include obesity, diabetes, cardiovascular disease, hypertension and stroke as well as some types of cancer."

Exercise

The need for physical activity was considered at the World Health Organization conference alongside diet. Panel members concluded:

- *Energy expenditures through physical activity determine body weight. Decreased physical activity contributes to the global epidemic of obesity.*

- *Physical activity has a great influence on body composition—on the amount of fat, muscle and bone tissue.*

- *To a large extent, physical activity and nutrients share the same metabolic pathways and can interact in various ways that influence the risk of several chronic diseases.*

- *Lack of physical activity is already a global health hazard and is a prevalent and rapidly increasing problem in both developed and developing countries.*

PREVENTING HEART DISEASE

The following risk factors have been associated with heart disease, and most are preventable:

Smoking

Smoking or being exposed to secondhand smoke causes several temporary effects in a person's heart and blood vessels. Nicotine in the smoke temporarily increases the blood pressure and heart rate. It also causes the arteries in the arms and legs to constrict and narrow. Although smoking doesn't cause high blood pressure, it increases the risk of developing cardiovascular disease in people with high blood pressure.

The carbon monoxide present in smoke is absorbed in the blood, reducing the oxygen available to the heart and to all other parts of the body. In addition, cigarette smoke causes clotting agents in the blood to become sticky and cluster. This shortens the survival of clotting agents, reduces clotting time, and makes blood thicker. Taken together, these effects harm a person's cardiovascular system.

Diet

When it comes to heart health, the foods that have received the most attention are fat and salt. Let's look at what we now know:

Fat
Of the four different kinds of fat, trans fat is the most dangerous, yet we rarely hear about this particular type of fat. There are four kinds of fats:

Monounsaturated fats (MUFA) are derived from plant sources, such as canola (62 percent), peanut (49 percent) and olive (77%). The benefits of monounsaturated fats include the following:

- Lowers the oxidation of LDL (bad) cholesterol slowing atherosclerotic plaque formation.

- Lowers triglyceride levels, a form of circulating fat found in plaque and cholesterol.

- Increases HDL (good) cholesterol, decreasing the risk of heart disease.

Natural Polyunsaturated Fats (PUFA) are considered to be a vital to our body's health. They are found in nuts, seeds and cold-water fish like salmon. While Omega-6 and Omega-3 PUFA found in soy oil, safflower oil, and sunflower oil are a healthy source of polyunsaturated fat; some PUFA oils have been commercially processed (see: "Unnatural Polyunsaturated Fat" below).

Unnatural Polyunsaturated Fats (PUFA) Although some polyunsaturated fats are healthy (those found in nuts and cold-water fish), some PUFAs are actually trans-PUFAs that have been subjected to destructive processes used to make oils. Manufacturers are allowed to print "high in polyunsaturates" on labels even though the product may be unhealthy. According to Udo Erasmus, who wrote *Fats That Heal Fats That Kill*, trans-PUFAs compete for enzymes, produce biologically nonfunctional derivatives, and interfere with the work of EFAs in our bodies.

Saturated fat, found in meat, poultry, butter, and milk, is only considered a bad fat in people with genetically abnormal LDL and HDL cholesterol levels. In people with normal HDL and LDL cholesterol, excess saturated fat is converted into monounsaturated fat, a good fat. Evaluations of fat in clogged arteries reveals that only about 26 percent is saturated. More than half is polyunsaturated.

Although saturated fats lower Lp(a), a substance that is associated with heart disease, the hormones and antibiotics that may be present in saturated fat are a major concern. Most saturated fat comes from animals reared on commercial farms where they are fed hormones to speed their growth and antibiotics to prevent diseases.

Trans fats are detrimental fats found in margarines, shortenings, and shortening oils. This type of fat impairs the cardiovascular system, the immune system, the reproductive system, energy metabolism, fat and essential fatty acid metabolism, liver function. and cell membranes.

The words *hydrogenated* or *partially hydrogenated* on product labeling indicate the presence of a trans fat, although sometimes this ingredient is not listed on food packaging. For example, Oreo cookies, made by Kraft/Nabisco, contain partially hydrogenated soybean oil, a trans fat. Although saturated fat must be listed on the "Nutrition Facts" label on food packaging, there will be no legal FDA requirement to list trans fat on the label until 2006.

So, in summary, good fats are essential to health.

Salt

Although salt has been linked to hypertension, Dr. John Laragh, of New York Hospital Cornell Medical Center—who is editor of the *American Journal of Hypertension*,—tells his patients to eat *unrefined* salt. In his research, he discovered that high blood pressure is caused by a hormone called renin and not salt (Note: the interactions between estrogens and the renin-angiotensin system are now being investigated). The salt he tells people to eat is not the bright white salt found in supermarkets but a gray salt that is sold in health food stores. When harvested from the sea and left in an unrefined state, unrefined sea salt has 88 minerals and *is always* light gray in color.

Refined iodized salt sold in supermarkets is a fraudulent food that is 99 percent sodium chloride with inorganic iodine added in the form of potassium iodide or sodium iodide. All macro and trace minerals that are present in natural salt have been removed.

Because human table-salt consumption comprises 7 percent of the total salt production, industry's demand for pure sodium chloride for the manufacture of chlorine, fertilizer, plastic, metallurgic, and atomic energy uses has driven salt manufacturers to create a cleaner, purer table salt devoid of all trace minerals. Dextrose is also added to stabilize the iodide compound in white table salt, and a bleaching agent is added to whiten an otherwise purplish powder.

It should be noted that salt used in processed foods (even brands sold in health food stores) is nearly always the refined commercial salt that is sold in supermarkets. Salt is a popular preservative because it binds with water and prevents the growth of bacteria that cause spoilage.

Cholesterol

The lipid hypothesis, as it is called, was introduced in the 1950s by University of Minnesota professor Ancel Keys. His hypothesis is that there is a direct relationship between the amount of saturated fat and cholesterol in the diet and the incidence of coronary heart disease. As strange as it sounds, Ancel Keys was recently interviewed by *Eating Light* magazine, and he said, "There's no connection whatsoever between cholesterol in food and cholesterol in the blood. And we've known that all along."

Although it is somewhat difficult to grasp what Ancel Keys recently had to say about the connection between dietary cholesterol and blood cholesterol, there have been a substantial number of studies contradicting the diet-cholesterol-coronary heart disease theory—it's just that we have not heard about them. One of the largest studies—now 55 years old—is the Framingham Heart Study under the direction of the National Heart, Lung and Blood Institute. Conducted in collaboration with Boston University, the researchers recruited 5,209 men between the ages of 30 and 62 from the town of Framingham, Massachusetts. Although Framingham study director Dr. William Kannel made the claim in the early 1980s that "total plasma cholesterol is a powerful predictor of death related to coronary heart disease," a decade later in 1992, the director—

Dr. William Castelli—admitted in an article published in the *Archives of Internal Medicine*:

> *In Framingham, Massachusetts, the more saturated fat one ate, the more cholesterol one ate, the more calories one ate, the lower the person's serum cholesterol...*

There is other evidence that is also difficult to fathom, given the pervasive promotion of "no cholesterol" or "low cholesterol" everywhere in the media. Let's look at the following facts:

- Although the consumption of saturated fat has plummeted, 40 percent of all deaths are from heart disease. From 1910 to 1970, the percentage of animal fat in the American diet declined from 83 percent to 62 percent. Butter consumption dropped from eighteen pounds per person per year to four.

- Dr. Michael DeBakey, who conducted the first successful angioplasty in 1954, the first coronary bypass in 1964, and the first heart transplant in 1968, told the *Washington Star*, "Much to the chagrin of my colleagues who believe in the polyunsaturated oil and cholesterol business, we have put our patients on no anticholesterol medications. About 80 percent of my 1,700 patients with severe atherosclerosis requiring surgery have cholesterols of normal people."

If you dig deeply enough, there is a vast amount of research all over the world to contradict the cholesterol-heart disease connection.

As we have seen in previous chapters, cholesterol is a building block for stress hormones as well as the sex hormones androgen, testosterone, estrogen, and progesterone. It is also a precursor to vitamin D and bile salts, and it is necessary for proper functioning of serotonin receptors in the brain. Recently, scientists have discovered that cholesterol is a powerful antioxidant that protects the body from free-radical damage. It is thought that high cholesterol levels in the blood reflect the body's need to protect itself from high levels of free radicals. Although there is probably no turning back for the American Heart Association, there are a growing number of medical professionals who now realize that the cause of heart disease is not animal fats and cholesterol but other dietary factors such as polyunsaturated (hydrogenated) fats, overconsumption of refined carbohydrates and sugar as well as vitamin and mineral deficiencies, particularly the antioxidants C and E as well as selenium, magnesium and iodine.

A growing number of cardiologists see heart disease as an inflammatory condition that can be detected early through the identification of correctable inflammation markers in the blood, including fibrinogen, homocysteine, and C-reactive protein. New research at the University of California at Irvine has found that high blood pressure can be induced—and brought back to normal—by changing levels of highly reactive oxygen molecules called free radicals. The study, which appears in the August 2003 issue of *Hypertension*, is believed to be the first to prove that increases in free radicals found in the diet can cause high blood pressure. The research suggests that multiple antioxidants in the diet, including vitamins E and C, may help prevent and treat certain types of high blood pressure.

PREVENTING OSTEOPOROSIS

Osteoporosis is largely preventable in most people. Bone is complex living tissue with nutritional and hormonal needs. At the present time, science is not certain how all of the nutrients needed to rebuild bone interact. There is much evidence that bone can be remineralized through hormone therapy and with prescription medication. Diet, exercise, and nutritional supplementation are important but have been disappointing in the fight to rebuild bone on their own.

Calcium

Of all the minerals needed to rebuild bone, calcium receives the most attention. Although calcium is an important element needed to build bone, there are many micronutrients needed to prevent osteoporosis. Calcium should never be taken alone but combined with vitamin K, folic acid, vitamin B6, magnesium, manganese, zinc, copper, boron, and silicon. Here are some important points:

- Calcium in doses of 600 to 1,500 milligrams per day is often recommended for the prevention and treatment of osteoporosis.

- Too much calcium may lead to a magnesium deficiency, which could accelerate osteoporosis; kidney stones are also a risk.

- Although there is no research establishing optimal calcium/magnesium ratios in the body, many practitioners recommend 2 milligrams of calcium for every 1 milligram of magnesium. Others recommend equal amounts and still others recommend taking twice as much magnesium as calcium.

- Inadequate calcium intake in adolescence will prevent a woman achieving maximum bone mass and will increase the risk of osteoporosis.

- The amount of calcium in your diet may be increased by eating calcium-rich foods such as milk, cheese, chickpeas, and broccoli. People who are lactose intolerant may have difficulty digesting dairy products because they lack the enzyme lactase, which is needed to break down the milk sugar lactose. Milk that is fermented with acidophilus is usually well tolerated in people who are lactose intolerant, as are yogurt and hard cheeses.

Factors That Upset Calcium Metabolism

While several vitamins and minerals assist in calcium utilization, there are several elements that upset calcium metabolism, including:

Sugar

Dr. Melvin Page, a doctor of dental surgery, studied bone loss in his patients and discovered normal calcium in their blood. He ran more than 2,000 blood chemistries and discovered that no absorption of bone occurred when the calcium and phosphorus ratios in the blood were in the ideal proportion of 10 to 4 (Note: Absorption refers to an erosion in bone that occurs when systems of the body need calcium). Page discovered that sugar upset the calcium/phosphorus ratio more than any other factor.

Lead and cadmium

Both of these heavy metals replace calcium in the bones, causing weakness and osteoporosis. Cadmium's toxicity also affects women's bodies in other ways. In *What Is Your Menopause Type?*, author Dr. Joseph Collins notes that the heavy metal cadmium is suspected of interfering with calcium's ability to increase steroid production, which could result in a decreased ability to convert cholesterol to pregnenolone.

Fluoride

Fluoride is also a heavy metal that replaces calcium in the bones. In the March 1990 issue of the *New England Journal of Medicine*, Mayo Clinic researchers published findings that fluoride increased hip-fracture rate and bone fragility.

Phosphorus

Phosphoric acid in soft drinks is believed to be a major cause of calcium deficiency in children and osteoporosis in adults. Too much phosphorus can upset the calcium-to-phosphorus ratio, causing calcium to be taken from the bones in order to correct it. This can lead to many of the problems of calcium deficiency, including osteoporosis.

Phytic acid foods

Phytic acid found in grains, beans, and soy is known to interfere with the absorption of crucial minerals, including calcium, magnesium, and zinc.

Oxalic acid foods

Oxalic acid found in spinach, Swiss chard, and chocolate combines with calcium to form calcium oxalate, a chemical salt the body eliminates.

Calcium from Food

The ideal way to take in calcium is through dairy products and bone broths. Small amounts of fine clay (sold commercially as bentonite) may also be added as a supplement to water or food—if it is very pure.

Dairy products

Dairy products are not only well-known sources of dietary calcium, but recent research suggests that they also help regulate body weight. A February 2003 article in the *American Journal of Clinical Nutrition* reviewed data from more than one human study showing a relationship between calcium and dairy intake to body weight. The studies showed that dietary calcium may play a role in regulating body weight; and increasing dietary calcium or dairy intake may help to curb future weight gain.

Dr. James Mercola, author of *The No Grain Diet*, describes an important distinction between pasteurized and unpasteurized, or raw milk. He explains that pasteurization destroys enzymes, vitamins B12 and B6, beneficial bacteria, and fragile milk proteins present in *real*, or raw, milk. According to Dr. Mercola, raw milk is an important whole food source that is available in 28 out of 50 states. Stores in California have started selling Organic Pastures's certified organic raw milk with colostrum, which recently received approval from the Department of Health Services (DHS) for the State of California. Colostrum is the first milk (actually a premilk) produced by the cow after giving birth and is a powerful immune system booster.

Dr. Mercola also recommends a Web site called realmilk.com which contains a list (organized by state) of companies that sell raw milk—www.realmilk.com/where2.html.

Bone broth

Bone broth (or soup stock) is full of bio-available calcium, magnesium, phosphorus, silicon, sulfur, and trace minerals. Bones from chicken, turkey, beef, or ham may be used. Add root vegetables such as turnips, parsnips and carrots, and simmer the broth for three to eight hours. Avoid sulfurous vegetables like cabbage or broccoli that can cause digestive upsets, and limit the cooking time for green vegetables to an hour or less to prevent bitterness.

Add a couple of tablespoons of vinegar, wine, or lemon juice to help draw the minerals from the bone and a large pinch of salt to help draw the juices from the vegetables. If you use uncooked bones, your stock will be white. Darker stocks that are preferred for winter recipes, are made from bones that have been roasted.

Calcium from Supplements

Although it is best to obtain a majority of daily calcium through your diet, it is not always possible. As a result, supplements help maintain the body's daily requirement for calcium. Here are some important facts:

Calcium carbonate vs. calcium citrate
The two most popular calcium supplements are calcium carbonate and calcium citrate. Although calcium carbonate is the cheapest calcium supplement, it requires high levels of stomach acid to dissolve. In truth, stomach acid is important for digestion and reducing it too much interferes with digestion.

Calcium citrate is a form of calcium that is far easier to absorb, does not require hydrochloric acid, and can be taken on an empty stomach. Because calcium has the potential to neutralize stomach acid, this supplement should not be taken with meals.

Calcium carbonate is also found in coral calcium, a popular new form of calcium that many experts feel is unsafe because of its aluminum content.

Elemental calcium on the label
The amount of calcium in your calcium supplement is labeled "elemental calcium." This number is usually one of two listed on the label. The other number lists total weight. Dr. Bess Dawson-Hughes, a professor of medicine at Tufts University and an expert on calcium, has explained it this way, "In calcium carbonate supplements, 40

percent of the total weight is calcium, and 60 percent is carbonate. This means that a 1,000 milligram tablet of calcium carbonate provides 400 milligram of elemental calcium. Calcium citrate, another commonly sold form, is about 20 percent elemental calcium."

Sugar and aspartame on the label
Beware of calcium candy called calcium chews. Cherry-and caramel-flavored chews contain not only sugar but many also contain hydrogenated oil and calcium carbonate, the most difficult calcium to absorb (see: "Preventing Heart Disease" for details about hydrogenated oils).

Supplements sold in pharmacies, discount stores, and supermarkets may contain ingredients such as sugar, starch, aspartame, artificial coloring, hydrogenated oil, and mineral oil, a petroleum product that has been known to block the absorption of fat-soluble vitamins.

Vitamin K

According to a study published in the *American Journal of Clinical Nutrition*, women who consume low levels of vitamin K have a greater risk of hip fractures than women who consume high or moderate levels of this nutrient. In a February 2003 paper published in the *American Journal of Clinical Nutrition*, researchers at the Jean Mayer USDA Human Nutrition Research Center on Aging at Tufts University showed that women with higher intakes of vitamin K had greater measured bone density than women with low intakes. The researchers found no connection between vitamin K intake and bone density in men.

Although vitamin K is available in green vegetables such as kale, spinach, and broccoli, new research suggests that postmenopausal women are not getting as much vitamin K as they need for bone health. Felicia Busch, author of *The New Nutrition*, recommends as much as 200 milligrams per day.

Because Vitamin K is involved in blood clotting, it blocks the action of blood thinning medications such as Coumadin, Heparin, and other related compounds. As a result, Vitamin K should not be taken by patients who take anticoagulants.

Vitamin D

Without vitamin D, you will be unable to absorb calcium from the foods you eat. Vitamin D is made from cholesterol molecules in the skin following exposure to sunlight and from fortified dairy products, egg yolks, saltwater fish, and liver.

It is estimated that 10 to 15 minutes exposure of hands, arms, and face to sun two to three times a week is enough to satisfy the body's vitamin D requirement. However, use of sunscreen and air pollution diminishes the production of vitamin D in the skin. As a result, nutritionists often recommend a daily intake of 200 to 400 IU per day.

Vitamin B6

As mentioned in the previous section, vitamin B6 is effective in reducing homocysteine, an amino acid thought to be a predictor of heart disease. According to Dr. Alan Gaby, author of *Preventing and Reversing Osteoporosis*, Vitamin B6 has been found to be deficient in people with hip fractures, and rats fed a vitamin B6-deficient diet developed osteoporosis.

Magnesium

Magnesium has proven to be effective in treating a wide range of conditions, including osteoporosis. Magnesium deficiency can inhibit vitamin D metabolism, which in turn can adversely affect bone building. Magnesium deficiency can also cause resistance to parathyroid hormone, which affects calcium balance, causing abnormal bone formation. However, it should also be noted that magnesium excess inhibits parathyroid hormone secretion, which also impairs bone metabolism. Although finding an appropriate calcium-to-magnesium balance is important in the prevention of osteoporosis, experts disagree over optimal calcium/magnesium ratios for supplementation. Many practitioners recommend 2 milligrams of calcium for every 1 milligram of magnesium.

Others recommend equal amounts, and still others recommend taking twice as much magnesium as calcium. Dr. Guy Abraham, a former professor of gynecology at the UCLA Medical School, favors a 2-to-1 ratio, or 2 milligrams of magnesium to 1 milligram of calcium. To test his hypothesis, he gave 19 postmenopausal women on hormonal replacement a supplement containing 500 milligrams of calcium (50 percent of RDA) and 600 milligrams of magnesium (200 percent of RDA) and did serial bone density studies every three months. Over a period of nine months, subjects receiving the treatment showed an 11 percent increase in mean bone density versus 0.7 percent in the untreated group.

Because calcium can collect in the soft tissues, we may appear to have a calcium deficiency when, in fact; we may have more than an adequate supply of calcium. This fact was illustrated in an experiment published by the *International Clinical Nutritional Review* in which volunteers on a low-magnesium diet were given both calcium and vitamin D supplements. All subjects were magnesium depleted, and although they had been given adequate supplements, all but one became calcium deficient. When given calcium intravenously, calcium blood levels rose, but only during the intravenous feeding. By adding magnesium, their magnesium levels rose and stabilized rapidly, and calcium levels also rose within a few days— although no additional calcium had been taken.

Hair analysis is thought to provide detail on the level of calcium in soft tissue, but it is highly controversial. Magnesium's ability to inhibit bone metabolism may be the reason many practitioners are more comfortable with a 1:1 ratio of calcium to magnesium.

Micronutrients

Several studies have shown the importance of micronutrients in preventing osteoporosis. The recommended daily dosage levels can often be satisfied by a high quality multiple vitamin:

Manganese
According to Dr. Alan Gaby, author of *Preventing and Reversing Osteoporosis*, food processing, coloring agents, preservatives, and

pesticides in our food, interfere with the absorption or utilization of manganese which can result in defective bone formation. He recommends supplements that contain 15 to 20 milligrams.

Folic acid

High homocysteine levels are considered to be a predictor for heart disease. Homocysteine also has a tendency to promote osteoporosis. At menopause, women are known to have a reduced capacity to metabolize homocysteine. Because folic acid is involved in the breakdown of homocysteine, it is considered to be helpful in preventing osteoporosis. Although the recommended dietary allowance of folic acid is .4 milligrams per day, levels used in studies to lower homocysteine have been as high as 5 milligrams per day. Women who take more than 1 milligram per day of folic acid should have a blood screening to test for pernicious anemia since folic acid may hide blood abnormalities associated with this disease, which is caused by a B12 deficiency.

Boron

In osteoporosis studies, boron has reduced the urinary excretion of calcium by as much as 44 percent. This may be because the synthesis of both estrogen and testosterone is enhanced by boron. As mentioned previously, testosterone promotes bone formation. However, testosterone excess can negatively affect the cardiovascular system and the insulin metabolism. Boron is often found in high quality multivitamins in very small doses of 1 to 2 milligrams. Women with excess testosterone should be careful about taking a multivitamin that contains boron.

Zinc

Zinc is known to enhance the action of vitamin D, which in turn enhances calcium absorption. Many high quality multivitamins contain 15 to 30 milligrams of zinc.

Copper

Because zinc interferes with the absorption of copper, it is thought that the potential for a copper deficiency exists if you take a zinc supplement. However, many people who have copper pipes may be absorbing copper through their pores when they shower. Foods rich in copper include whole grains, leafy green vegetables, nuts, eggs, and poultry.

Protein

Although protein intake has been thought to promote urinary excretion of calcium because of the need to buffer the acidic breakdown products of protein, researchers have also speculated that protein intake may increase bone density. In a study published in the April 2002 issue of the *American Journal of Clinical Nutrition*, subjects over 65 years of age who ate high protein showed improved bone mineral density measurements, but only in those patients also taking calcium and vitamin D supplements.

Weight-Bearing Exercise

Bone becomes stronger and denser when you perform weight-bearing and resistance exercises. For example, tennis players typically have a bigger and denser bone in their playing arm than they do in their other arm. This can be confirmed through X-ray. Weight-bearing exercises are those in which your bones and muscles work against gravity. Examples include jogging, walking, stair climbing, dancing, and soccer. Resistance exercises are activities that use muscular strength. Examples include weight lifting and using weight machines found at gyms.

PREVENTING ALZHEIMER'S DISEASE

Although Alzheimer's is an incurable, progressive, terminal brain disease that afflicts mainly the elderly, numerous risk factors have been identified:

Aluminum

Autopsies on Alzheimer's victims have revealed excessive amounts of aluminum in brain tissue. Aluminum is a popular metal used to make pots and pans and beer, soda, and other food cans. It is also found in antacids, baking powder, buffered aspirin, pickles, antiperspirants, deodorants, bleached flour, table salt, tobacco smoke, cream of tartar, Parmesan and other grated cheeses, and processed cheese. Studies have shown that in the presence of fluoride, aluminum leaches out of cookware. Boiling fluoridated tap water in an aluminum pan leached almost 200 parts per million of aluminum into the water in ten minutes.

Fluoride

In October of 2002, research by the National Institutes of Environmental Health Sciences (NIEHS) reported that fluoride has synergistic effects on the toxicity of aluminum. Most drinking water contains a substantial amount of fluoroaluminum complexes. According to the NIEHS report, most water treatment processes result in increased levels of aluminum in the finished drinking water. The report stated that fluoridation will result in aluminum fluoride compounds that enhance neurotoxicity.

Vitamin and Mineral Deficiencies

The following vitamins and minerals have been shown to help Alzheimer's disease patients:

Choline

Alzheimer's patients have a deficiency of the neurotransmitter acetylcholine because they are deficient in the enzyme choline acetyltransferase. The result is a decrease in the amount of acetylcholine in the brain. A study performed in the 1970s demonstrated that the brains of those with Alzheimer's disease contained 60 to 90 percent less of the enzyme choline acetyltransferase than did the brains of healthy persons. Increasing dietary choline raises blood and brain levels of acetylcholine. Choline is readily available in lecithin.

Calcium and magnesium

Calcium and magnesium have been shown to slow down aluminum

absorption. These minerals also play an important role in the prevention of osteoporosis.

Antioxidants

Alzheimer's patients have abnormally low measurable levels of vitamin E and carotene in their bodies. Antioxidants have been thought to slow down or prevent Alzheimer's disease.

Vitamin B12

Recently published research indicates that Alzheimer's disease might be related to deficiencies in vitamin B12 and folic acid. It is thought that the possible mechanism for these vitamin deficiencies leading to Alzheimer's disease might lie in their relationship to homocysteine. A deficiency of either vitamin B12 or folate can lead to higher homocysteine levels in the blood, and homocysteine has damaging effects on the central nervous system, leading to such diseases as Alzheimer's.

Vitamin C and tyrosine

The neurotransmitter norepinephrine, considered to be helpful to Alzheimer's disease patients, is made from the amino acid tyrosine, which is made from phenylalanine. Like other amino acids, phenylalanine is derived from the meat in our diets, but the conversion to tyrosine requires vitamin C.

PREVENTING CANCER

Numerous observational studies have shown beneficial effects of both foods and nutrients that break down carcinogens in the body.

Cruciferous Vegetables

Laboratory studies show that cruciferous vegetables such as cabbage, cauliflower, brussels sprouts, and radishes contain a number of cancer-fighting substances, including indole-3-carbinol (I3C). Indole-3-carbinol stimulates the rate at which the body eliminates estrogen through a pathway known as the tumor suppressor pathway or 2-hydroxylation. Indole-30-carbinol has been shown to be an effective weapon against breast, cervical, and skin cancer.

Cruciferous vegetables also contain phytochemicals called isothiocyanates, which stimulate the body to make enzymes that break down carcinogens.

Asparagus

The anticancer property of asparagus comes from an antioxidant called glutathione, which has been found in animal studies to inhibit tumor growth. Asparagus also provides almost 33 percent of a day's requirement for folic acid, which has been shown to lower cancer of the cervix, colon, and rectum (see: "Folic Acid").

Alliums

Alliums are a group of vegetables that includes onions, garlic, leeks, chives, scallions, and shallots. These vegetables are rich sources of organosulfur compounds, or OSCs, that have been shown to have anticancer properties. OSCs are good at protecting against DNA damage caused by carcinogens, particularly of heterocyclic amines, which are formed in the high heat cooking of meats.

Tomatoes

Tomatoes, preferably uncooked, are full of lycopene, which helps prevent lung, colon, prostate, and breast cancer. In one study, elderly Americans who ate a diet high in tomatoes had 50 percent fewer cancers overall than those who did not. Animal studies have also found some cancer-preventative benefits with lycopene.

The deep red color in tomatoes that is also present in watermelons, red peppers, and guavas is caused by lycopene, a carotenoid that acts as a dietary precursor to vitamin A. Lycopene is a very powerful antioxidant. By donating its electrons to free radicals, lycopene neutralizes them.

Other Disease-Fighting Nutritional Elements

The following nutritional elements are promising disease fighters:

Vitamin C

Nobel prize—winning Linus Pauling, Ph.D. and Ewan Cameron, M.D., a Scottish cancer surgeon, demonstrated that ten grams of vitamin C a day reversed terminal cancer in 13 out of 100 patients.

Folic acid

Studies show that people who get higher-than-average amounts of folic acid from their diets or supplements have lower risks of colon cancer and breast cancer.

Antioxidants

Oxygen-scavenging free radicals that are produced from an internal process of oxidation are extremely unstable particles that damage the outer protective membranes of cells. Although they have been implicated in more than 60 disorders, including heart disease, cancer, Alzheimer's disease, cataracts, and rheumatoid arthritis, free radicals also serve a beneficial function in helping to kill invading pathogens, thereby preventing inflammation.

Vitamins such as A, C, and E are powerful free-radical scavengers. These are found in most fruits, vegetables, and whole grains. One of the most powerful, pycnogenol, is highly present in pine bark and grape seeds.

Glutathione

Dr. John Pinto, of the Memorial Sloan-Kettering Cancer Center in New York, calls glutathione, the master antioxidant. Jean Carper, in her book *Stop Aging Now!*, says, "You must get your levels of glutathione up if you want to keep your youth and live longer. High levels of GSH [glutathione] predict good health and long life. Low levels predict early disease and death."

Glutathione is the body's universal antioxidant. Many protective systems of the body, including those that use vitamins C and E, depend heavily upon this protein, which is produced naturally in the body. The body actually performs a form of chelation on heavy metals (cadmium, lead, mercury) with glutathione. A healthy liver will produce a backup supply of glutathione when supplied with sulfur, found in foods such as asparagus, garlic, onions, and eggs.

CONCLUSION

▼

The purpose of this book is to help women make important decisions about their own health. By providing factual information to improve their skills in interpreting risks and benefits from the results of widely publicized studies, I hope many women will feel more comfortable with the choices they have made. I spend many hours a day caring for and educating patients about the often-confusing health information available to them. If I have succeeded in the book's purpose, I hope I will have performed a service for my generation.

About the Author
Carol Uebelacker, M.D.

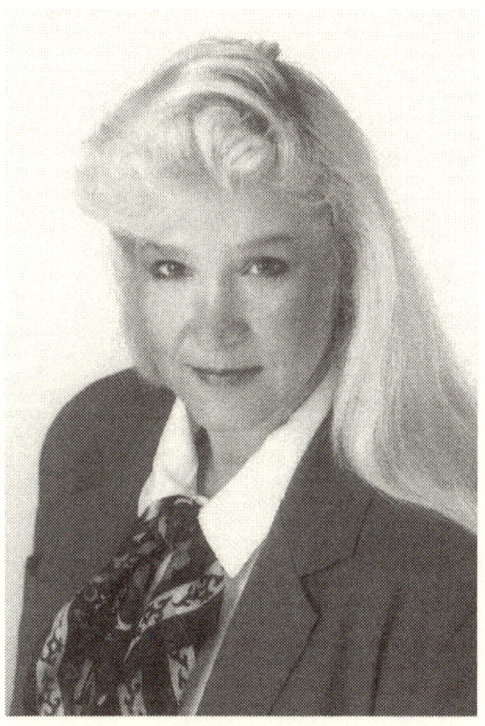

Carol Uebelacker is a board-certified family physician who has been practicing in Delafield, Wisconsin, since 1991. Her specialties include women's health and alternative medicine. She is a graduate of the University of Wisconsin Medical School in Madison, Wisconsin, and completed a family practice residency at the Hinsdale Family Practice Residency Program in Hinsdale, Illinois. She is a fellow of the American Academy of Family Physicians, a member of the State Medical Society of Wisconsin, the Waukesha County Medical Society, the Milwaukee County Medical Society, the Wisconsin Academy of Family Physicians, and the American College for the Advancement of Medicine.

In 2002, Carol served as president of the Waukesha County Medical Society. She has served on the State Medical Society's Council on Mediation and Peer Review as well as the Executive Committee of the Waukesha County Medical Society. She has been a guest speaker in many public forums, covering topics such as menopause, women's health, smoking cessation, and common pediatric problems.

Index

0-595-30878-3

www.ingramcontent.com/pod-product-compliance
Lightning Source LLC
Chambersburg PA
CBHW020248290526
45784CB00003B/1146